## STUART M. BERGER, M.D.,

received his medical degree from Tufts University
and is a graduate of the Harvard School of Public
Health. A specialist in nutritional medicine with a
private practice in New York City, he is the author
of two previous bestsellers, including *How to Be
Your Own Nutritionist,* and a popular *New York
Post* column. In 1987 he received the State University of New York's George W. Thorn Award for
extraordinary professional accomplishment.

*Other Avon Books by*
**Stuart M. Berger, M.D.**

HOW TO BE YOUR OWN NUTRITIONIST

*Coming Soon*

FOREVER YOUNG

# WHAT YOUR DOCTOR DIDN'T LEARN IN MEDICAL SCHOOL

## Stuart M. Berger, M.D.

AVON BOOKS ◆ NEW YORK

AVON BOOKS
A division of
The Hearst Corporation
105 Madison Avenue
New York, New York 10016

This book is dedicated to all my patients who have had trust and faith in me and the vital importance of nutritional medicine. These patients have demonstrated the need for medicine to become more consumer-oriented and, by demanding the use of preventive care in health, have begun to change the traditional outlook of medicine as it is known today.

# Acknowledgments

A special acknowledgment to Pat Golbitz, Sherry Arden, Howard Kaminsky, Larry Hughes, Allen Marchioni, and Rena Wolner, who represent publishing at its best.

And to those friends and associates whose advice and devotion have sustained me through the joys, as well as the difficulties, of achieving what I've set out to do. Among them are Lorna Darmour, Arthur Klebanoff, Marlaine Selip, Marilyn O'Reilly, Oscar and Marion Dystel, Frank and Jackie Devine, Roger and Pat Wood, John Mack Carter, Walter Sabo, and Sally and Karl Soderlund.

A special acknowledgment to my friend and colleague, David Nimmons, who is responsible for writing this book, and his research assistant, Charlene Laino.

With love to my parents, Rachel and Otto, who exemplify how corrected nutrition helps overcome critical medical conditions. Their enduring support will always give me strength. And in loving memory of my Uncle Harry.

# Contents

# One Patient's Story,
# or Why I Wrote This Book

This book properly takes its beginning in the year 1976, when I was completing my medical training. I was working as a resident at New York University Medical Center when a woman came in to see one of the breast surgeons there. Frightened about a growing lump in her breast, she had gone to see her family doctor. He told her to see a surgeon as soon as possible and referred her to one of the cancer surgeons at the hospital. Unfortunately, the specialist was so busy that she had had to wait two months to get an appointment. Somehow, she managed to control her mounting terror as she felt the lump grow larger and larger, not even daring to talk with her family about the problem. When the surgeon finally saw her, the news was doubly grim: Not only was it cancer, but no bed was available in the hospital for four to six weeks.

It was at this point that she telephoned me. I listened to her story, and behind it, the deep fear in her voice. Was there really no choice, she pleaded? I found it hard to believe myself—after all, every day on the surgical wards I saw patients admitted to the hospital for elective procedures, minor hernia operations, plastic surgery—yet for a woman who could die from her disease, she could have no operation for six weeks.

I placed a call to a friend of mine, Dr. William Cahan, an eminent surgeon at the world-renowned Memorial Sloan-

Kettering Cancer Center. I finally tracked him down on a Friday night, weekending with friends in the Hamptons, ninety minutes away from Manhattan. "Bring her out tomorrow morning, and I'll examine her at the cottage." He was as good as his word, and after the examination, he turned to us. "This cannot wait. I want her admitted to Sloan-Kettering tomorrow." She was, and the following day, this master surgeon successfully operated to remove the tumor.

But the woman's story was far from over. Because the cancer had spread in her chest, she was referred to another doctor to begin an intensive course of chemotherapy. The deadly drugs would have been agonizing enough, but the procedures of the chemotherapy clinic made it worse. They demanded payment in cash before each treatment. "After all," they explained, "with cancer patients, well . . . we have to collect up front." I could scarcely believe that a system could be so degrading, so stressful, sending patients such a defeatist, pessimistic message; but rules, they told me matter-of-factly, were rules.

After several months of the anguishing drug treatments, the chemotherapy doctor noticed an imbalance of liver enzymes in one of the woman's routine blood tests. He ordered an X-ray scan. It brought bad news: an unidentified mass on her liver. He was blunt, and pessimistic: "The cancer has probably spread. Your only chance for survival is the most aggressive chemotherapy possible." It was almost too much for the shattered woman to bear. Just when she saw an end in sight to her painful ordeal, she was instead beginning another.

Her second round, I knew, would be much worse. Chemotherapy drugs in those days worked by literally poisoning the patients to the very precipice of death, and then doctors tried to bring them back. Too often they failed. In her case, they would pump her full of a devil's cocktail of the most toxic drugs known to medicine, drugs that would damage her organs, damage her own defenses, even unleash their own cancerous changes in her body. She would spend months vomiting, nauseated, weak, unable to walk or eat. The drugs would chemically eat away and destroy her adrenal glands completely, in hopes of arresting the cancer in her liver. I saw this brave woman, who had faced everything so far with courage and grace, begin to doubt that she would make it through this next round. Tears in her eyes, she asked me, "Isn't there really . . . any other choice?"

She had only two days before she was scheduled to begin the chemical treatment, so I recommended one other expert. His approach was straightforward: "Operate first. I'd want to know there was definitely a tumor there before she takes a drop of chemo."

On his advice, exploratory surgery was done, with stunning news: The "mass" was a simple, benign cyst, which she had most likely had since birth. And, it turned out, the chemical imbalance that had so alarmed the chemotherapy doctor turned out to be due, not to a new cancer, but to the very chemo drugs she had been taking.

I was in her hospital room when she heard the news. As the news sunk in, she started to tremble. She had come only days away from being pumped full of the most lethal, debilitating agents—drugs quite capable of crippling or even killing her—for a cancer she never had. Today, ten years later, that same woman is alive and in robust health. I know, because that patient was my mother.

If the medical system had taken a slightly different course, she might well not be here today. Her life could have been forfeited to delay, mismanagement, the needless toxic interventions of a medical system run amok. I also know that the same is true of every man, woman, and child who participates in our medical system—and that means all of us. This sorry state of things is a simple fact of American medicine, one that holds true for you, for your loved ones, and for your friends. The truth is that *we are all at risk simply because of how our medical system functions.* Or, to put it another way, because of what our doctors didn't learn in medical school.

But it doesn't have to be this way. Each one of us, given proper information, intelligence, and a cooperative physician, can greatly improve our own medical odds. We can learn to make the system work with us, for us, increase and improve our own health and that of those we love. Most important of all, we can learn to avoid the powerful ways that our medical system and its illness-centered view of medicine keeps us unhealthy, makes us sick, and actually raises our risk of medical problems.

If you hear a resonant ring of truth here, and if you have ever found yourself wondering if there isn't a better way, then you are the person I am writing this book for. I hope you'll find something to take away with you in the pages that follow.

# 1

# The Breakdown of the Medical Machine

I consider myself lucky. Early in my medical career, I had a ringside seat at a major medical foul-up. Having watched the medical system fail so spectacularly, and at such close range, with someone I love so much as my own mother was a lesson I have never forgotten. Since that day, I have never been able to believe with the same confidence and enthusiasm that our doctors and hospitals, our drugs and devices, will always create a happy ending, or that practitioners of the medical arts are assured of healing and healing well. A week does not go by that I am not grateful for that skepticism.

I have become acutely aware of the patients whose lives have been irreparably damaged, whose faculties and families have been shattered, because they fell between the cracks of our medical system. I have seen even more suffer with handicaps and serious chronic medical problems that are entirely unnecessary—because of what their doctors didn't know.

Like most of my practicing colleagues, I have seen up close that even the best doctors, in the best institutions, using the best technologies and tools available, don't always create the best outcomes for patients. To this day, I cannot look at my mother without knowing that she—in fact, my father and my entire family—very nearly became medical victims.

Nearly losing my mother to the excesses of medicine

gone mad was a wrenching experience for a young and impressionable medical student. I began questioning inside, examining what I was learning to do and be in this arduous medical training. I began wondering what else I was being taught that they didn't really understand. I recall looking over at my classmates during one grand rounds and worrying, Are we just learning to accept a whole system of medically approved blind spots?

In many ways, I knew, I was extremely lucky. After all, I was doing my medical apprenticeship at the finest institutions: Tufts Medical School, Harvard School of Public Health, New York's prestigious University Hospital, and the psychiatric wards of Bellevue Hospital. My classmates and I had access to the finest medical minds, the most advanced space-age technologies: digital analyzers, ultrasound probes, electron-scintillation cell counters, microprocessor-based life-support devices, scores of different computers. We learned to interpret more than five hundred sophisticated lab tests and assays, we witnessed and performed death-defying surgical techniques and mastered complex skills of machine-assisted life support. In those days, in the excitement and rush, we had little time to stop and reflect or to ask the obvious questions: We were learning immense amounts—but were we learning what we should? We were becoming doctors, to be sure, but were we becoming better healers?

I soon found myself beginning my internship, the brutal rite of passage that tempers all physicians. Every doctor knows the terrified feeling of showing up on the wards the first day, knowing he or she is expected to help people, but not having the first clue as to how. I had never taken a pulse, inserted a catheter, sutured a wound, drawn a blood sample, even taken an accurate history. Neither I nor my classmates knew even the rudimentary skills of doctoring. We were expected to learn as we went, on the run, using our patients as human workbooks. In theory, older doctors were there to guide us; in the grim practice of the wards, we were on our own, left to fend and figure as best we could.

## The Thirty-Six-Hour Nightmare

For every physician, those years of internship and residency hold agony and terror. You can work shifts of thirty-six hours, handle all-night on-calls, see your personal and emotional life become utterly and totally destroyed.

My own experience consisted of a blur of twenty-two-hour days of exhaustion. Although it happened some dozen years ago, I still recall vividly the night I was awakened from sleep at 3:00 A.M. I was needed—immediately—at the hospital, because they had an accident and needed every available hand. Never mind that I had been working for the previous thirty-six hours or that this two-hour slice of sleep was all I had to prepare me for my next twenty-four-hour rotation, beginning at 4:00 A.M. Wondering if I was being pushed over a precipice of human endurance, I got up, threw a lab coat over my pajamas, stumbled into the street, and started to walk the two blocks to the hospital.

Feeling myself about to collapse, slipping on the icy Boston sidewalks, bleary-eyed with fatigue, I hailed a passing cab. When I said, "Emergency," I am sure the driver thought I was an ailing patient, not a physician. Trembling, soaked with perspiration, I fairly fell through the doors of the emergency room. I can't imagine that the sight of this unshaven, disheveled intern could give anyone confidence—I surely looked worse than many of the people I was there to treat. As I entered, the head nurse looked up: "What took you so long? It doesn't matter anyway—Dr. Levine took care of it. We don't need you." Stung with anger and guilt, I stumbled out into the snow, feeling tears on my cheeks.

Every practicing doctor I know has a very personal version of this story. We recount them not to glorify ourselves, but because they give a glimpse of our system of "macho medicine," which trains its healers by driving them to the brink of madness.

Any doctor who has been through it knows that the thirty-six-hour system is as much a nightmare for patients as it is for doctors—and it is absolutely no way to deliver decent care. Consider this brief—and telling—dialogue between a reporter and a doctor on a national news program:

REPORTER: Are you going to care for a patient as well in your thirtieth hour as you did in your third hour on duty?

PHYSICIAN: Definitely not. People are much more forgetful, less attentive to detail, less able to concentrate after that kind of sleep deprivation.

Another medical colleague chimed in with his story: "I remember being here for thirty-six hours straight, no sleep . . . too tired to even think. The quality of medical care would improve with shorter hours . . . you'd much rather have somebody at four o'clock in the morning when you're having chest pain who's alert and oriented and had not been up for a long time. It's just common sense."

A third doctor told an even more alarming story: "I've seen thirty-four hours continuously nonstop, and that's about as far as I can go. Somewhere around twenty-four hours is where you start to cry, and somewhere before that you might hallucinate now and then."

(At long last, just as this book was going to press, the health commissioner of New York State just announced a new ruling—no more thirty-six-hour shifts for medical interns. Why? Because a young woman was killed in a New York hospital when she was admitted into an emergency room and received "woefully" inadequate care at the hands of interns and residents working unsupervised thirty-six-hour shifts. But although one state may have come to its senses and removed this most glaring flaw in our medical system, forty-nine states have not tackled the problem at all. In those states—probably *your* state—the thirty-six-hour nightmare remains the rule for doctors learning medicine . . . and their unfortunate patients.)

Through those endless days and nights of our training process, we knew something was very wrong—but we never had the time to ask what. We were so concerned about packing in all the information we were given, mastering the overwhelming rush of data and facts, knowing how to put the pieces together, that it never occurred to us that there might be things we were neglecting altogether.

Even then, there were hints and clues. During my residency, I noticed that patients I visited in the hospital sometimes seemed to respond less to my treatments and medicines than to a moment of my time, my arm laid on theirs, or simply a kind and cheering word. Clearly they were starved for it. Prisoners in beds, confined by their sickness to a scary and unfamiliar world, they were pumped and poked and prodded and probed, yet what they needed most of all was someone to listen, someone to take a moment, someone to care. But there was no time for that—it was not on the curriculum, not a part of the program. I found myself asking where compassion and humanity were taught, but the fact was, we were being trained as doctors, not healers, and they weren't always the same thing.

The system believed it was important that we know how to drive a sharp, hollow needle (trocar) into a person's living chest without anesthetic in ten seconds in an emergency room, but never taught us how to help our patients live so that they would never be brought into that emergency room. We learned how to use scalpels, deadly drugs, and radiation beams to destroy cancer, but not how the right food and life-styles could help prevent cancer in the first place.

After my training, I opened my own practice, in the heart of New York's busiest, most exclusive borough.

Every day my waiting room filled with desperate, despairing people. Many feel they have exhausted all their options, that they really have no place else to turn. They complain of a whole range of chronic, debilitating symptoms, yet have been unable to find out why they have them. By the time they reach me, they often feel powerless and worried, watching their health and mental stability erode.

They are veterans of the medical mill, and in their charts I see a wake of puzzled doctors, ineffective treatments, and mountains of medical bills. Yet they have not yet won relief from the amorphous symptoms that weigh them down, degrading their health and their lives. Universally, I notice, they feel out of control and frustrated, desperate to get a grip on their failing health.

Whatever the complaint that brings them to my waiting room, these people are smart, motivated, and medically sophisticated—yet the medical system is letting them down. They don't need a medical quick-fix, but a way to take control of their own health and well-being. Yet, at every turn, they find themselves running up against a system that denies them the help they need to stay well, reinforces them for getting sick, and whose powerful tools often make their conditions worse instead of better.

These people don't need wonder drugs, crash programs, or the crazy prescriptions of the latest health fads. What they *do* need is a way to break the sickness cycle, see through the hype and the obfuscation, and learn how to get—and keep—themselves as healthy as possible.

Daily, I watched the steady procession of these patients, people who didn't need to be sick. Many had the resources to avail themselves of the best medical care possible. I realized that they represented a shocking defeat of what I had been taught in medical school. They had simply slipped through the cracks of the medical machine. The more I treated their long list of symptoms, complaints, and problems, the more I realized they were a living indictment of the way we do medicine. They are—and I have no kinder term for it—victims of our institutionalized medical ignorance, the case studies of what their doctors don't know.

## An Ounce of Prevention

The supreme irony is that many of the cases I see are, to a great extent, preventable. Those people, and millions like them, suffer from diseases that didn't ever have to happen. They lead twilight lives, frustrated, disabled, and depressed, because their conditions fall outside the high-tech expertise of modern medicine. Lives are wasted, even lost—because our physicians are not trained to recognize and cure certain kinds of complaints. In later chapters of this book, we will examine more deeply the kinds of diseases that most commonly fall between the cracks of our American medical system. They are as varied as they are profound: thyroid problems, hypoglycemia, immune dysfunction, chronic fungal infections such as candidiasis, the wide range of premenstrual disorders, occult food sensitivities. We'll discuss not only the signs and symptoms, and how you can tell if you may be affected by them, but equally important, why they get overlooked by our medical system.

I really do hope that you will take away from this book something far more valuable than an abstract discussion of our medical system: You'll learn a series of ways to make the medical system work better, be more responsive—and responsible—to you. You'll gain an understanding of specific medical problems that may be affecting your life, happiness, strength, and well-being, and that may have gone unnoticed. More important, we'll focus together on what you, as an individual, can do about them.

I see people with these problems every day at my office. I am continually reminded that if our system were truly one of prevention and health, instead of reaction and illness, there would not be so many people waiting in my—or any other physician's—waiting room. But until recently, the medical and scientific minds who drive our system have not paid due attention to aggressively preventing illness. For all of us, whole areas of preventive health remain largely uncharted, and the discoveries they promise for longer and better health go untapped. In short, our medical myopia sentences millions of Americans to anguish, poor health, even premature aging and death.

Take such a basic, commonsense area as nutrition. All of us learned in grade school about the four basic food groups. But the advances we have made since then would leave your grade-school health teacher absolutely amazed. No longer are we confined to a murky notion of the "four basic food groups." Nutritional science has undergone a true revolution, and modern clinical nutritionists, and their colleagues in the laboratory nutritional sciences, are many times more sophisticated and knowledgeable. We now have real, proven means to delay or prevent health problems such as cancer, heart disease, vascular problems, various psychological disorders, and a host of other medical emergencies. Yet that knowledge is not moving out of the laboratory to help patients in need. Why not?

Of the 127 medical schools in this country, only 24 of them—fewer than 20 percent—require courses in nutrition. Of the top 15 medical schools, only about one-quarter offer such courses. Think of the message that sends to the prospective physician: In 1987, they are still four times more likely to attend a school where they don't have to take a course in preventive nutrition than one where they do.

The situation is even worse when it comes to the field of preventive medicine. Only one medical school, the University of Rochester, now requires a full-fledged course in preventive medicine; in all the nation, only two other schools even ask their students to devote a single medical clerkship rotation in the field of prevention. In the other 98 percent of medical schools, prevention is taught as an afterthought, between the lines—or, most often, in no systematic way whatsoever. Is it any wonder that our nation spent $425 billion on medical care last year?

The real question is: How much of that colossal bill—not to mention the uncountable human suffering it represents—came from diseases that could have been prevented in the first place? In recent congressional testimony, former secretary of Health, Education and Welfare Joseph Califano estimated that 67 percent of the diseases we now treat could have been prevented. That would mean we spend over $250 billion each year to treat needless, preventable diseases. In 1985, the Public Citizens Health Research Group issued a paper estimating that over $100 billion is spent every year for preventable diseases. Another $100 billion, they wrote, is spent for unnecessary surgical procedures. For one disease such as high blood pressure, which is largely preventable, Americans will spend more than $10 billion this year. What the experts seem to agree on is that fully 50 percent of our massive medical outlays are wasted—spent for illnesses we should not have had to begin with and for operations we don't need. Clearly, the simple, sane idea of prevention has gotten crushed beneath the wheels of the billion-dollar medical juggernaut.

## Something Old, Something New

But a lack of preventive knowledge isn't the only problem. Another real consideration is the impossibility of physicians' keeping themselves abreast of the torrent of new medical information they must know. This has become enough of a problem that medical educators around the country have recognized it. One of my favorite quotes comes from Dr. David S. Greer, dean of medicine at Brown University, who told a recent graduating class: "Fifty percent of what we have taught you is wrong. Our problem is that we don't know which fifty percent."

If this is a difficulty for medical students, it is a huge problem for real-life doctors. The age of the average practicing physician in this country is forty-seven years old. That means that Dr. Average attended medical school about twenty years ago—back in the Middle Ages in terms of medical innovation. Twenty years ago, there was no such thing as gene-splicing, artificial hearts, or test-tube *(in vitro)* conception. Devices such as laser scalpels, fiber-optic surgical scopes, and Nuclear Magnetic Resonance Imagers did not exist. Now-common drugs such as beta-blockers for the heart, the many so-called ''rational'' drugs, and revolutionary developments such as artifical blood would not be created for many years. Monoclonal antibodies, the tiny chemical keys that have opened doors to understanding AIDS and cancer, were not even conceived of in research laboratories. The very idea of substances that can boost or build the immune system—what we know of today as the promising immune modulators—seemed pure science fiction. The list is endless, and a testament to the pace of medical progress.

But where does that leave Dr. Average? Since many of these tools and techniques came along after he—and most of the practicing physicians out there—had completed their formal training, they never had the chance to learn about these complex technologies and tools thoroughly, comprehensively, and accurately. James S. Todd, deputy executive vice president of the American Medical Association, summed up the problem succinctly: ''In terms of procedures and drugs of major benefit, doctors generally learn of their existence rather quickly. But they may not really learn how to use them in the most effective manner possible.''

As I was writing this chapter, the American Association for the Advancement of Science convened a seminar addressing the fact that even the most highly trained radiologic physicians are falling behind the stunning technological advances in radiology. They conclude, ''Advances in radiology technology may be outpacing users' ability to interpret the data provided.'' It's a scary thought—that our machines' competence has outstripped our own. Surely, if our radiology specialists have such problems, what about the general internists and family doctors who were trained long before such advances even existed on the drawing board?

But it is not just technology that is changing. At a more profound level, there have been fundamental biological breakthroughs in our understanding of hormones, cell biology, cancer, neurotransmitters, and a host of other crucial physiological processes, that practicing doctors may not even ever fully learn about.

The problem is worse for older doctors—the large percentage of them who are in their fifties, sixties, even seventies. When they trained, we did not know about DNA, had no polio vaccine, no effective cancer chemotherapy, no cardiopulmonary resuscitation, and the field of cell biology did not even exist. We had not yet invented the cardiac pacemaker, electron microscopes; the first open-heart surgery had not been done; and the most basic pharmaceutical tools in our arsenal against mental disease—including the whole range of antidepressant drugs and tranquilizers—did not yet exist.

I do not mean to suggest that only youth or book learning makes a good doctor—that would be both false and presumptuous. The most inspirational medical mind I ever met was one of my professors at Tufts, who was then in his early seventies. His encyclopedic knowledge of diseases and symptoms made him a superlative diagnostician, renowned for his acumen and insight.

The same point was brought home to me recently when a friend recounted the story of taking her three-year-old child to a very old country doctor. She had been home in the rural farm town where her parents live when her son fell sick. What first seemed a minor bug soon grew worse. As his fever climbed to 103, she could see that he was getting weaker and weaker—but, isolated in the country, there was nobody to turn to except the now-venerable GP, who had treated her thirty years ago. The visit to his tiny office confirmed her worst fears; the doddering physician seemed barely able to hear her. Intently, the aged doctor listened to the child's chest, thumped and prodded, and took a careful pulse. As he stood up, he smiled and patted the child's head. Shakingly, he wrote out a prescription: "This ought to help," he shouted. Desperate, she saw no other choice and gave the medicine to her son. Within a few hours, the fever broke. For the first time in days, her son slept sweetly, his breathing easy. I have no idea what miracle medicament that old doctor prescribed, but he proved the maxim that the best medicine is often as much art, learned by experience, as science, learned at school.

But, while experience counts for much, it is not enough. It cannot keep pace with the innovation and progress of our massive medical-knowledge industry. Regardless of the breadth of a physician's experience, it is today humanly impossible to keep truly current and informed on more than a fraction of the new developments, technologies, and treatments entering the medical system.

The American Medical Association has estimated that there are sixteen thousand medical journals being published today. Even if a physician were to read only those directly related to his or her specialty, it would be more than a full-time job. With biomedical knowledge currently doubling every eight years, the gap between a doctor's knowledge and the state of the art is a chasm that no doctor can fully bridge. Of course, it is not just academic knowledge that is growing so fast: The AMA estimates that 30 to 40 percent of the average physician's procedures and diagnostics have been developed in the last decade alone.

As though to underscore the point, I just picked up this week's *New England Journal of Medicine* and find myself reading about what could be a tremendous research breakthrough—a simple blood test that can diagnose cancers with 90 percent accuracy. Two months ago, this test didn't exist. Last year, it would have been considered fantasy. Who knows what tomorrow's medical headlines will promise? The fact is, in a very real way, what your doctor didn't learn in medical school is most everything—and as we all know, what your doctor doesn't know *can* hurt you.

## Caught in the Medical Machine

Given the deluge of new information, and with so many doctors who finished their medical training years ago, the American medical machine suffers from serious built-in obsolescence. Even as our most conscientious doctors run in place frantically trying to keep up, every year they slip further and further behind. The result is that, in the world's most complex and "advanced" medical system, you as a patient are forced into an insidious choice: An older doctor who offers you the wisdom of experience, or a younger one with a more thorough knowledge of the newest advances. This double bind keeps patients and doctors alike stuck on the medical treadmill.

You may assume, as many patients of mine do, that physicians are supposed to keep their knowledge current. In fact, that rule is honored as much in the breach than in the observance. In 60 percent of this nation's states, physicians don't have to take a single hour of instruction after they get their licenses. Even in the two out of five states that do require ongoing education, the standards are often ludicrously low. As every doctor's family knows, it is possible to attend a seminar in Honolulu, register one's name each morning, lie on the beach all day for three days, and pass one's continuing-education requirement for the year. I am not suggesting that most physicians do this; most of the doctors I work with are dedicated and sincere, and devote a huge amount of time to keeping their knowledge current. But if they keep up, they do so almost in spite of the system—certainly not because of it.

There is the same laxity in board certification. Many physicians are certified in a medical specialty—psychiatry, cardiology, obstetrics, pediatrics, or the like. But, in many of those specialties, once you pass the original certifying exam, you won't be required to take another test—ever.

And the specialties that do require you to prove your continuing knowledge only require an exam every seven or ten years. A lot can happen, and a lot of patients can be hurt, in a decade.

The whole topic of recertification has become highly politicized. In most specialties, only the newest doctors have to submit to recertification. Those who were already practicing when the rule went into effect—and that means most of the nation's practitioners—are exempt. Thanks to a "grandfather" provision, those physicians have won themselves a lifetime tenure in their specialty—no holds barred, no questions asked. It is both surprising and disturbing that only two specialties—family practice and emergency medicine—require all their members to recertify their knowledge. In the twenty-one others, a board-certified doctor who passes a test at age thirty-one can hold the same certification at age eighty-one—and nobody will ask a thing.

On the one hand, we have an overwhelming crush of new medical information, on the other practitioners who have scant time to master it and a system with few checks to make sure that they do. So how does that affect you when you go into your doctor's office? Clearly, patients and practitioners alike worry about the changing face of medicine. Doctors' offices, once sanctuaries of reassurance and personal contact, have become assembly lines of forms, insurance, and procedures. Everybody knows the experience of having a doctor who's busy, unable to return your phone calls quickly. One new patient disgustedly told me of the arrangement her last doctor followed: He'd answer phone questions from patients only between 3:15 and 3:30 on Tuesdays and Thursdays. If you didn't happen to be sick then or couldn't get through—too bad.

## Beyond the Problem

What we will do in these pages is look more closely at why things are as they are, not from the point of view of an academic medical expert, but from the point of view of you, the person in your doctor's office. You will see specifically what kinds of diseases and disorders are most often overlooked, so that you can help yourself if you think they may be affecting you.

Most of all, we will work together to give you the tools you need to cooperate with your doctor, within the system, to make it work for you. If you are tired of being out of control when it comes to your health, tired of being swept along in the medical maelstrom—bobbing, catapulting, and eventually being left high and dry—this book holds some useful information.

# 2

# Caution: Doctors May Be Hazardous to Your Health

*"I die by the help of too many physicians."*
—Alexander the Great, 323 B.C.

Over the many months I spent researching and writing this book, one experience kept occurring again and again. Perhaps I was attending a reception, a professional meeting, or just dinner with friends, when somebody asked what I was writing about. When I explained that I was writing about the problems in our way of doing medicine, and what people can do to overcome them, the response was always the same: "Problems with the medical system? That must be a very thick book!" Whether they are patients, friends, other professionals, or just acquaintances at large, everybody agrees: Something is very wrong with the American pursuit of health. The secret is out that our nation's way of healing is sick indeed.

I don't believe there's any one simple cause for this state of affairs. In my experience, it is not usually due to ineptitude or incompetence on the part of doctors or health professionals. If it were, that would be much easier, because then we would just have to weed out the bad ones from the good.

But that's really not the case. Most physicians I know are conscientious and well-meaning. They try as best they can to deliver good care, to guide and support their patients, helping them through the medical maze to health.

But they are frustrated. Doctors, like those we treat, are mired in the same difficult system, squeezed by the same counterproductive rules and procedures, constrained by the same assumptions. *All of us, patient and practitioner alike, are caught in a vast, expensive, elaborate medical machine, one that very often works against our health and well-being.*

What I want to do is to invite you along with me to give the American medical establishment its own "checkup," a sort of physical to see where it is faltering. Together, we will don a physician's white coat and stethoscope. We will prod and poke American medicine in its vitals, look together at how things really are, and try to peel back the gleaming facade of modern, high-tech medicine, to reach the very human struggles beneath.

What are we up to here? When physicians seek to understand a patient as a whole, we often examine just a part. A biopsy reveals the nature of a larger growth; from a drop of blood we extrapolate the body's chemical equilibrium; taking your pulse can reveal the health of the whole cardiovascular system.

In much the same way, I think we can get a good idea of the health of our overall medical system by focusing on several distinct areas within it. By themselves, they are not complete nor exhaustive, but together they give us a good idea of how well our health care system is working to keep us healthy and make us well when we're not.

The first principle of the Hippocratic Oath, to which every doctor must swear before he or she can treat patients, reads, *"Primum, non nocere* (First, do no harm)."

This first principle—so basic, so evident—ought to be absolutely incontrovertible. Yet equally certain is the fact that many times each day in this country, it is blatantly violated. For this, too, doctors have coined an appropriately Latinate word: *iatrogenesis.* Behind this fancy, three-dollar term, spoken in hushed tones within the medical priesthood, is a simple idea: the diseases and sickness caused by doctors (*iatro*, doctor, plus *genesis*, created). Obviously, it refers to more than just doctors; it includes nurses, hospitals, drugs, vaccinations, chiropractors—any regiment of the healing armies that, in fact, make a condition worse or create another one.

Few people appreciate just how widespread such diseases are. If you think for a moment, you may realize you have been affected yourself. Have you had a bad reaction to a drug the doctor prescribed? Been confined to bed for a day after a routine flu vaccination? Endured complications from surgery or childbirth? If so, you are a firsthand iatrogenic victim.

How common are these diseases? Unbelievably so. In a letter in the prestigious *New England Journal of Medicine*, one physician writes that for every patient that medicine is able to dramatically help, there is one patient who is in some way harmed. This doesn't include the vast majority—eight out of ten, according to this particular author—who have things that either get better on their own or that doctors don't know how to help much. Taken on the whole, he writes, "The balance of accounts ends up marginally on the positive side of zero."

## An RX for Risk

Perhaps the most widespread way our medical establishment makes us sick comes through the drugs we take. It was the great physician Oliver Wendell Holmes who wrote, "A medicine . . . is always *directly* hurtful; it may sometimes be indirectly beneficial. I firmly believe that if most of the pharmacopaeia were sunk to the bottom of the sea, it would be all the better for Mankind and all the worse for the fishes." Unfortunately, in some ways those words are as true today as they were when he wrote them. In the last half century, there have been several epidemics due purely and simply to unforeseen drug reactions.

In 1937, the antibiotic sulfanilamide was marketed dissolved in a lethal liquid: Scores of people sickened and died. In 1942, hundreds of troops who received a yellow-fever vaccine contracted potentially deadly hepatitis B; in 1955, an epidemic of polio was traced to an incorrectly prepared vaccine; five years later, the tragic epidemic of birth defects among women in several countries taking thalidomide; in 1971, a wave of hospital patients contracted lethal sepsis from intravenous fluids contaminated with bacteria. In all these cases, the problem was not that people were incorrectly taking these medicines—but that the drugs they trusted for their health had serious toxic problems, were incorrectly prescribed, or had some serious unanticipated effects. They were made sicker by the careful ministrations of our medical machine.

In recent memory, there have been two particularly tragic instances where people were hurt by what their doctors didn't know about the drugs they prescribed.

In one of the most publicized cases, 2.6 million expectant mothers in the United States took the drug DES to help prevent miscarriages. But in 1971, doctors at the Massachusetts General Hospital discovered that many of the children born to those women were developing vaginal cancer. Looking more deeply into it, it turned out that up to 7 percent of DES daughters developed signs of such cancers. In addition, sons born to mothers who had used the drug have a higher rate of cancer of the testicles. The mothers themselves have a greatly increased rate of breast cancer. The story is doubly tragic, because several studies also show that the drug doesn't significantly lower the risk of miscarriage. But because of what doctors didn't know about that drug, experts estimate that of these women, "well over 80,000 of them now have cancerous or precancerous changes of their reproductive organs attributable to . . . DES, and that more will develop them as they get older."

How many people remember reading the news headlines in 1982, about a new drug called benoxaprofen. In that year, the FDA licensed the drug, the first of a new kind of nonsteroid drug that arthritis patients could take once a day to relieve their debilitating joint inflammation, pain, and stiffness. But four short months later, it was taken off the market, when British authorities revealed that sixty-one patients in that country had died from complications of the drug. Although it worked to reduce pain and arthritis symptoms, it also created lethal liver and kidney damage—a fact that was not observed in the testing in this country. Happily, this drug was caught before there were any such needless deaths in our country, but the fact that it ever slipped through our screening system in the first place points up the inadequacy of our safeguards.

It is comforting to think that such stories are a problem of the past. Comforting, but wrong. Last year, the Food and Drug Administration estimated there were some forty thousand such drug-induced episodes in our nation. The vast majority don't kill people, but they can cause suffering, cost money, and require or lengthen hospital stays. And, of course, some do cost lives.

One study of patients in a Pittsburgh medical center tracked the number of drug accidents in one intensive care unit over a five-year period. There were ninety-two instances of human error and fifty-three cases of machine malfunction. The result for the patients was significant: Those who experienced adverse drug reactions were only half as likely to leave intensive care alive.

For every adverse drug reaction we know about, many go unreported. Many doctors and hospitals don't keep track of these occurrences. But perhaps more should. One study at a Minneapolis hospital found that, when they started logging bad drug reactions for the first time, incidents rose from one per year to thirty in four months! And in a particularly telling glimpse into hospital practices, they admitted, "This is not a large number for an institution of our size." Figures like this explain why, in 1986, more than two decades after the thalidomide tragedy, an English researcher wrote, "The number of patients injured or killed in epidemics of drug-induced disease is a vast multiple of the number of thalidomide victims; the range of injuries produced is also so wide that no simple solution to the problems is likely to emerge.''

The solution is clearly more complex than Dr. Holmes's suggestion of a century ago, but until then, all of us should remember that the drugs we swallow, inject, inhale, and apply every day have their own built-in flaws—part of the hidden price we all pay for our way of healing. They are the harvest of what we forgot to teach in medical school.

## The Hazards of Hospitalization

''Hazards'' is not a word we usually associate with hospitals. We tend instead to view a hospital as a palace of care and nurturance, an oasis where we go to be rescued from the trials of illness and accidents. Unfortunately, in the way the medical establishment currently works, that is far from the case. In fact, the ''hazards'' title of this section comes from the titles of two separate research papers appearing within three years of each other in different medical journals. One was from Yale Medical School, the other from the University of North Carolina. Together, they pointed out a fact most doctors know only too well: that these temples of medicine are also laboratories for creating illness.

Does this sound like an exaggeration? I wish it were. Consider these statistics:

• A Yale University study twenty years ago showed that 1 patient out of every 5—20 percent who was admitted to a teaching hospital suffered an iatrogenic episode. Two decades later, a similar study was reported in the *New England Journal of Medicine*. Instead of decreasing, the number had almost doubled: Of 815 people admitted to one hospital's wards, over one-third (36 percent) were hit with a doctor-caused illness. In a quarter of those, the problem was grave enough to threaten life or produce ''considerable disability.'' Two people out of every hundred died from them.

- Research from Boston, reported in the *American Journal of Medicine,* looked at over a hundred patients who developed serious kidney problems while hospitalized. Of those, over half were thought to be caused by procedures and treatments in the hospital, including X-ray dyes, restricted blood supply, and kidney-damaging antibiotics.
- The *American Journal of Epidemiology* recently reported that about 6 patients in every 100 admitted to hospitals will contract some kind of infection, one they didn't have upon admission. The researchers estimated that as many as 4 million of these infections may occur each year. Based on that figure, it means that 108,000 people will die—either entirely or in part due to the infections they acquired courtesy of the medical machine.

I recall one day in medical school, shortly after I began making rounds on the wards, having a sinking revelation: that hospitals, just like any other human enterprise, are just a vast interlocking constellation of human foibles, frailties, and failings. People screw up, confusion abounds, politics fester, neglect occurs, greed persists. Things are, in short, no different than in a corporation, a neighborhood, or a Girl Scout troop. The stakes are just higher.

This fact explains the most glaring of the hospital hazards, and the one you probably thought of first—negligence. These cases are as tragic as they are dramatic: the eighteen-year-old girl with a high fever who dies because a young intern in the emergency room gives her a drug that reacts with medicine she is already taking; the young man who is brought to the hospital in an acute asthma attack, whom nobody examines for twenty-five minutes, so he suffocates; the feverish child "with a flu," given aspirin and sent home from the hospital, where she dies of undiagnosed meningitis. I wish I could report that these are fictional cases, but they're not; each of them, and forty other equally serious cases, occurred in the last three years in my own city, New York—arguably the city with the world's most advanced, intensive medical system.

Such tragedies can, and do, happen anywhere, on a more or less daily basis, in hospitals around the country. While terribly tragic and grim, they are the result of the machine breaking down—people not doing what they should, forgetting, being careless. And though these negligence cases make the most dramatic headlines, they are, in some ways, the easiest to prevent.

Far more serious are the problems that are built into the system, that are in fact intrinsic to how the medical machine functions. They are usually more subtle, harder to pin down and eliminate, and less likely to change. It is those, not the well-publicized cases of negligence, that put us at greatest risk.

## High-Tech, Yes—High-Safety . . . Maybe

Recent medical progress has brought dramatic advances in methods of diagnosis and treatment. With each new advance, however, reports of adverse reactions have soon followed. The occurrence of occasional reactions is now considered to be an accustomed and almost predictable hazard.

Those words were written by a professor of medicine at Yale University in 1963. Since then, the rate of medical progress has more than tripled—and with it, the rate of unforeseen hazards. In the intervening years, the problem has gotten worse, not better, as our medical enthusiasm for intensive, invasive procedures, made possible by high-tech developments, creates its own malaise in our medical practice.

Sadly, the mania for high-tech gizmos seems sometimes to have more to do with concern for appearance and modernity for its own sake than with serious medical judgment. A few years ago, a colleague of mine had just returned from medical study in Oxford, England. She recounted a furious debate then raging among the physicians at Oxford's prestigious teaching hospital: Should they acquire another CAT scanner, at a cost of over a million pounds? As the debate grew heated, one of the most eminent senior professors arose and asked, "Let us consider how much extra skilled nursing care we could buy with a million pounds. Wouldn't that improve quality of care far more?" I recall marveling at that sentiment, because I knew just how unheard-of such a remark would have been in my own country at the time. The point was brought home again recently when I read an article quoting the president of one of the nation's largest hospitals talking about those same CAT scanners: " 'We need one because they have one' can be the biggest factor," he explained. That difference, I believe, categorizes much of why we are where we are.

## Deadly Diagnostics?

No area has grown faster—or has accrued more technology—than the field of diagnosis. We have developed an array of staggering new technologies, including Nuclear Magnetic Resonance Imaging, fiber optics, ultrasound, cardiac catheterization, and angiography. These, and a host of other sci-fi, high-tech technologies, have changed the face of diagnosis. But some procedures that patients may view as relatively harmless can have serious—even fatal—side effects.

Look at where we are today:

Researchers at the renowned Walter Reed Army Hospital studied hospital patients for eight years and recorded 125 cases of doctor-caused injuries to blood vessels severe enough to require immediate surgery. *Two-thirds came from diagnostic procedures.* Some of the hapless patients even suffered more than one serious injury at the same time! All told, these medically induced accidents resulted in two deaths, four amputations, and eight people left functionally disabled. In their discussion, the physicians highlighted a disturbing trend: Between 1966 and 1968 only 10 such cases occurred at the hospital. By 1982, after a decade of "progress" and more invasive diagnostic procedures, the hospital reported 13 cases each year—an increase of more than four times.

A similar study in the *Archives of Surgery* reported on patients at a Texas teaching hospital who suffered significant blood-vessel injury. Among the forty-six patients with iatrogenic injuries, *more than half* were due to diagnostic procedures.

Among the procedures that can create problems are endoscopic examinations of various organs and procedures such as coronary angiography, where doctors take pictures of the heart vessels. Even common X rays, at radiation levels previously thought to be benign, have been recognized to carry significant health consequences.

One of the most space-age of the new medical technologies is the growth of high-intensity-beam electron and X-ray therapy for tumors. Many modern medical centers today bristle with the most sophisticated electron and X-ray accelerators, huge ray guns that zap tumors. But while there is no doubt that these have saved many, many lives, they have also taken some. Last fall, the *American Medical News* reported three injuries caused by a state-of-the-art X-ray machine. Instead of the usual therapeutic dose, these patients received a dose *125 times higher* than usual. One, a woman from Georgia, escaped with the loss of her left breast and a permanently disabled left arm; tragically, both of the men—one just thirty-three years old—died of the injuries they received at the hands of our high-tech medical establishment. The error was traced to a computer "bug," an error in the computer program controlling the machine.

## A Nosocomial Nightmare

Most of the ways we create illness in our medical system have little to do with computer "bugs." They concern the much more ordinary kind of "bugs," such as the lowly bacteria, viruses, and parasites we catch every day. Unfortunately, they abound in the very places where the medical practitioners ply their trade: doctor's offices, clinics, operating theaters, and hospital wards. They abound in such profusion, in fact, that the medical priesthood has coined a term for them, *nosocomial infections,* the infections you acquire in the clutches of the medical system.

The hospital into which you place yourself for the best care teems with hundreds of different germs that can make you sick. One researcher, from Case Western Reserve Medical School, laid it out in a recent article in a medical journal:

> By its very nature, a hospital is a veritable reservoir of bacteria. Any time an already sick, weakened patient is exposed to an environment and personnel that harbor a variety of virulent bacteria, the risk of infection is increased. In addition, today's hospital contains within its walls not only increased numbers and types of microorganisms, but also hard-to-treat, newly resistant pathogens.

In other words, checking into the hospital is like jumping into a pool swarming with infectious piranhas—and you're the bait. It is, to borrow the medical parlance, a nosocomial nightmare.

Such infections represent the single largest chance that a person undergoing medical care is likely to contract an iatrogenic disease. These agents—*pathogens* is the medicalese—may be diminutive, but the problems they cause are anything but. As I already mentioned, about 6 patients out of 100 admitted to hospitals will acquire some infection they didn't have when they came in. For more than 100,000 people this year, those infections will cause, or contribute to, death.

The most recent estimate from scientists at the Centers

for Disease Control indicate that if you are a patient undergoing surgery at many of our largest teaching hospitals,
you run a risk of one in seventeen of having your convalescence complicated by a significant infection. Even in
local hospitals, your risk is about one in twenty. If you
are one of the unlucky ones, catching such an infection
means you may remain in the hospital up to five days
longer, spending an average of $355 per day extra on your
hospital bills. And, of course, each extra day you stay in
the system, the more likely you are to contract another
infection. It's a built-in, self-perpetuating cycle that un-
dermines health and sabotages well-being.

In one recent year, public health authorities surveyed a
small percentage of the nation's hospitals. Yet even in their
tiny sample—just fifty-four hospitals—they counted more
than twenty-eight thousand medically induced infections.
In that study alone, people contracted infections of the
urinary tract, respiratory tract, lungs, blood, surgical in-
cisions, and skin.

The problem is hardly confined to hospitals. You may
have a parent, family member, or older friend or relative
who is in an extended-care or nursing facility. These people are also at risk. According to one study, which inves-
tigated nearly all the nursing homes in the state of
Arkansas, tuberculosis was so endemic that people's risk
of contracting the disease rose in direct proportion to how
long they had lived there. High rates of infections have
also been found at veterans' homes. In total, nosocomial
infections cost us about two billion dollars each year in
prolonged hospital stays alone.

Such infections range from irritating rashes to life-
threatening blood and organ infections. To take just one
of these, consider the situation with the serious liver disease, hepatitis A. In one recent six-year period, studies
have traced at least thirteen outbreaks of this highly infectious liver disease to hospitals.

What happened in Lexington, Kentucky, was typical.
Doctors in a hospital's newborn ward gave blood transfu-

sions to eleven babies, all from one single unit of blood. A week later, they learned that the blood—all from one donor—was contaminated with a case of hepatitis that was undiagnosed when the donor gave the blood. Not only were those eleven babies infected, but it soon spread to three other babies in the nursery. Next, the virus showed up among some of the doctors and nurses. Finally, the liver disease moved out among the newborns' parents, siblings, and families. By the time it was over, fifty-five people, in several states, had been infected. As the physicians noted, with no apparent sense of irony, the newborns' intensive care unit "appears to be ideal for the transmission of hepatitis A." There is a wider lesson in this example, one that I find highly disturbing. Those fifty-five people, countless others in the other dozen outbreaks of hepatitis A, and millions of others across this nation, contracted a serious and costly disease that never should have happened. Each is an iatrogenic victim, a case study of our medical establishment doing precisely the opposite of what it was intended to do.

The ways our medical machine transmits illness is a model of efficiency. On instruments, hands, clothing, hitchhiking germs on nurses, orderlies, and doctors—even the air in many medical settings can transmit sickness. In one three-year-period, a British team found twenty-four cases where outbreaks of *Salmonella* poisoning in hospitals were caused by contaminated food served to the patients. If you have ever been hospitalized, you know that hospital food has long been a joke. But it is not a joke at all when such food actually makes patients sicker. It would seem that if people are in enough trouble to be hospitalized, the least the hospitals could do is avoid poisoning them with the food once they're in.

## The Dirt on Doctors

I think the most unsettling fact is that many of these infections are, quite simply, avoidable. Perhaps the most stunning recent indictment was reported in the *Journal of the American Medical Association*. In the study, which was as simple as it was scandalous, researchers simply counted how often medical personnel wash their hands between patients.

It was in the mid-nineteenth century that British surgeon Joseph Lister pioneered the idea of antiseptic surgery, and the famed Hungarian obstetrician Ignaz Philipp Semmelweiss instituted the practice of washing hands and using sterile procedures in childbirth. That means that for more than a century physicians have known about this basic precaution, the most elementary of all safeguards— a low-cost, easy, effective way to minimize infections. Yet this study suggests that modern physicians have somewhat forgotten the early lesson of Lister and Semmelweiss. Their findings are truly shocking: "On average, hospital personnel washed their hands after contact with patients less than half the time. Physicians were among the worst offenders." Need we ask how many of the billions of dollars—not to mention the suffering of thousands of people—could be avoided by this simple safeguard? Nobody knows.

The lesson of the doctors' dirty hands holds true on a larger scale, as well. The fact is that we already have protocols and procedures that can reduce many of these life-threatening infections. Doing so is, in reality, no great mystery. Epidemiologists and biostatisticians have clearly shown that hospitals that institute strict regimes can reduce the frequency of nosocomial infections by about one-third. But, sadly, only a small percentage of hospitals have instituted the broad-based programs they should. Experts estimate that, as recently as the 1970s, only 6 percent of such infections were being prevented. If all our hospitals were to adopt those procedures today, we could cut the rate by 26 percent. Instead, they don't, and the rates of these infections continue to climb. I cannot help wondering if a few less Magnetic Resonance Imagers and a few more bars of soap wouldn't be a sound investment in our nation's health.

Deadly drugs, dangerous diagnostics, rampant infections, slipshod procedures—clearly, the best thing you can do for your health is to stay as far away from hospitals as possible.

But staying away is not as easy as it sounds. Indeed, one of the most insidious forces of the medical machine is its tendency to put too many people on a conveyor belt to the very hospitals where they run a high risk of being made sicker. This is usually done in the name of delivering the most care to the most people. But what we need to realize is that the most care is not necessarily the best care, especially given our proven ability to make people sicker. As one researcher wrote, "The possibility of too much medical care and the attendant likelihood of iatrogenic illness is presumably as strong as the possibility of not enough service and the attendant morbidity and mortality." Translation: Doing too much hurts people as much as doing too little.

Yet still the machine goes on, drawing people to our hospital doors like a vast, irresistible magnet. Study after study has shown that a shockingly large proportion of admissions to hospitals are simply unnecessary. The most recent research comes from the Rand Corporation, reported in the *Journal of the American Medical Association*. Their verdict? About one person in four who is hospitalized may not need to be. When they include people who could just as well have been treated as an outpatient, instead of in a hospital, the number leaps to 40 percent. What all of those people may not know is just how they are risking their lives unnecessarily as they sign their admission forms.

Researchers have cited this pattern of needless hospitalization again and again:

• A survey of federal employees showed that more than half of the operations they underwent could be classified as unnecessary—fully 53.5%.

- Among members of two New York unions that were studied, about *one-third* of the women had hysterectomies that didn't need to be done.
- According to an independent study reported by the Senate Committee on Aging, up to one-half of the cardiac pacemaker implants that Americans undergo are unnecessary—the result of overaggressive treatment and people not getting second opinions.
- Researchers at Cornell Medical School had 1,356 patients who had been recommended to undergo major surgery reexamined by board-certified specialists. The specialists found that fully one-quarter of the recommended operations—one in four—was not needed. In some surgical specialties, it was even worse. In orthopedics, more than 40 percent of the recommended surgeries were judged unnecessary; in urology, over one-third.

Although the specific numbers may vary, the trend is clear (see the illustration on page 32). Too often the old surgical adage "When in doubt, cut it out" is being followed all down the surgical line: gall bladder removals, hernia procedures, appendix operations. What is less clear is that we are helping anybody when we do so.

## The Unkindest Cut of All

Almost all of those needless visits boil down to one word: surgery. There is little more puzzling in our way of healing than how we commit surgery—or, more correctly, how *often*. It is puzzling primarily because it seems to flaunt one of our basic axioms. For if there's one first principle on which everybody ought to agree, it is that any operation is a dangerous thing, one to be avoided if at all possible.

In the most recent year for which we have statistics, 1985, Americans underwent almost thirty-seven *million*

## PERCENTAGE OF POTENTIALLY NEEDLESS SURGERY BY BODY PART

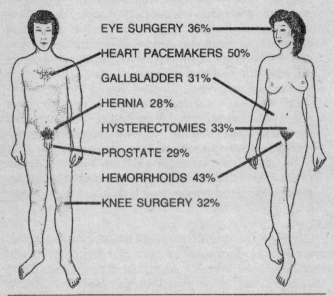

EYE SURGERY 36%

HEART PACEMAKERS 50%

GALLBLADDER 31%

HERNIA 28%

HYSTERECTOMIES 33%

PROSTATE 29%

HEMORRHOIDS 43%

KNEE SURGERY 32%

surgical procedures, says the National Center for Health Statistics. A recent congressional report found that over the last decade rates of surgery increased four times faster than the population grew. Behind those statistics is a very real change in all of our lives: For you, and everybody you know, the statistical chances you would be put under the knife rose four times! Another, more conservative study found that rates of surgery "only" went up 93 percent in the last decade—effectively doubling our chances of winding up on an operating table.

Of those, it is impossible to know how many were truly necessary, but it is clear that it is far from all of them. A decade ago, when Americans underwent exactly half as many operations as we do today, experts testified before Congress that more than three million operations each year were unnecessary. Today, twice as many people go under the knife—a 100 percent "surgical inflation"—which puts the number of needless, endangering procedures at about six million each year. That's six million times when people put their lives at risk, either from the operation itself or from the iatrogenic circus surrounding it.

In terms of dollars, that waste is staggering. The Public Citizens Health Research Group estimates that we spend more than $10 billion each year on surgical procedures that didn't have to happen in the first place. A study in the *New England Journal* article examined sixteen patients at one hospital—patients who had problematic colon operations. Had all gone smoothly with their operations, these patients would have been expected to stay in a total of 235 days; instead, their complications kept them in 984 days, four times as long. Instead of the combined bill of approximately $94,000 that one would project, their total bill was $670,000—seven times as much.

But more worrisome than the dollar value is the human cost, and that we can never measure on paper. Two years later, these same authors looked at another group of thirty-six patients who suffered from serious errors in surgical care. Twenty of the thirty-six never left the hospital, and for more than half, death was "directly attributable" to the surgeon's error. Of the sixteen survivors, almost one-third left the hospital with some serious physical disability. In total, of the thirty-six studied, less than one-third of the patients had a satisfactory result from their surgery. On a national level, the figures grow even more tragic. Even the most conservative figures suggest that some twenty-five thousand people lost their lives as a consequence of needless surgery last year. Their names should be added to the growing list of iatrogenic victims, but no such memorial exists. Instead, they are memorialized in the hearts of families and friends, who are left wondering, "What happened?"

When the surgical stakes seem so high, and the reasons

to avoid them so clear, why does our medical establishment guide so many people into the hospital and under the knife? In this, as in many facets of American medicine, the closer you look, the more confusing things become.

If you're like most people, you tend to trust that you'll get operated on when you should; that is, if you have such-and-such a problem, you'll get such-and-such treatment. It sounds neat and tidy in theory, but in practice it doesn't work that way. Research suggests that, for any one of us, whether you get put in the hospital, and what will happen to you if you do, depends on factors much more arcane and mysterious than simply what you may have. Your zip code, for example.

- In a now-classic study, a researcher at Dartmouth Medical School determined that a woman is 80 percent more likely to undergo a hysterectomy if she lives south of the Mason-Dixon Line than if she lives in our northeastern states. One can't help but suspect that such figures reflect more about attitudes held by southern male physicians about their female patients than about any biological reality. That idea is supported by a Canadian study showing that when an independent state agency began to monitor how often hysterectomies were performed, the rate dropped by half!
- In one area examined, seven out of ten children had their tonsils out by age fifteen; among similar children in another region, more than nine in ten still had their tonsils *intact.*
- Iowans suffering from heart disease are twice as likely to have open-heart surgery if their address is in Des Moines than if they live one hundred miles away in Iowa City. Californians with the same diagnosis would have a two-thirds higher chance of coming under the surgeon's knife if they lived in San Diego than if they lived a day's drive up the coast, in Palo Alto.

* Residents in some areas in Kansas are four times as likely to undergo any elective surgery than people living in other regions of the same state. What seemed to account for the wide variations? The number of board-certified surgeons in a given region.
* The likelihood that hernia patients in Massachusetts will have an operation varies almost 400 percent from one part of the state to the other; for their neighbors seeking heart pacemaker operations, the rate among different cities in that state varies over 1,000 percent!

So what does this variation really mean? Why does it matter? Among all the figures, it's easy to lose sight of the human facts behind the statistics. But one researcher put it into perspective. He noted an immense variation in the rate of prostate-removal surgery among different regions. Then he sat down at his calculator and asked a simple question: What would happen if we did prostate surgery at the *lowest* regional rate versus the highest regional rate? His startling conclusion: We would save fully five thousand lives each year!

## Schedule Your Sickness?

Just as where you live has an effect on your care, so does when you get sick. Researchers in Pittsburgh found clearly that the most drug-related accidents in the wards—wrong prescriptions, improper dosages, incorrect or dangerous administration—occurred in those same months of July and August, exactly when the new doctors, residents, and nurses, new to hospital procedures, first arrived on the wards.

I recently saw a news broadcast in which a medical resident put into words what every physician who trained in a major teaching hospital knows. "July is a very dangerous month in the hospital. Everybody is new. They don't know their way around the hospital . . . and they don't necessarily know what they're doing."

Clearly, in a medical establishment that practices "diagnosis by zip code" and "treatment by calendar," something is very wrong—and very dangerous.

## The Best Medicine Money Can Buy?

One can't help but wonder what other nonsensical factors may also conspire to make us such an overhospitalized, overoperated-on people. Perhaps the best answer to that was given fifty years ago, by Dr. Richard Cabot, professor of clinical medicine at Harvard University.

In 1938 he said:

> The greatest single curse in medicine is the curse of unnecessary operations, and there would be fewer of them if the doctor got the same salary whether he operated or not. We would never put a judge on the bench under conditions such that he might be influenced by pecuniary considerations. Suppose that if the judge were to hand down one decision, he got five thousand dollars, and if he decided the other way, he got nothing. But we allow the private practitioner to face this sort of temptation. To have doctors working on salary would be better for doctors as well as for patients.

Fifty years later, his words still hold true. When it comes to surgery, the free-market principles of supply and demand create a paradox: There are simply too many people in whose interest it is to subject other people to surgery.

The United States has twice the number of surgeons, per capita, as does, say, England or Wales. With so many willing hands on the market, it should come as little surprise that American surgeons also perform twice as many operations. According to those statistics, joked one of my patients, an insurance statistician, we all have an easy way of cutting our risk of surgery in half: move abroad!

For prospective mothers, that advice is particularly well taken. Thanks to the functioning of our medical machine, a woman is more likely to deliver her baby by caesarean section in this country than in any other country on earth—including Britain, Canada, and France. In part that is due to the U.S. medical doctrine—never proven—that once a woman has had her first baby by C-section, she has to have her next that way, too. I am not convinced that research supports this rule, but with so many surgeons around, I don't see obstetrical practitioners lining up to challenge it.

When it comes to the surgeon glut, perhaps the most radical solution was offered more than a decade ago by an unlikely source. The former president of the American Medical Association, Dr. Walter Bornemeler, wrote, ''Just chop the number of surgical residencies in half, and in about ten years, we'll have just the right amount.''

Surgeons would have us believe there is little financial incentive in their decisions to operate, but even a quick look at the figures suggests otherwise. The fact is, study after study shows that doctors in HMOs (health maintenance organizations), who work on salary, order fewer routine X rays and electrocardiograms and perform fewer caesarean sections, coronary bypasses, and general surgery than do doctors who get paid for each operation. Certainly, such patients are being exposed to less surgery risk. But in the long run, are they suffering from this lack of operations?

No, according to one scientist at Harvard Medical School. Dr. Thomas Graybois looked at one hundred patients who were candidates for open-heart, coronary bypass surgery. These were not the sickest, critical-care patients but those for whom the life-threatening operation was elective. Seventy-six of them declined the operation—and seventy-five of those were still alive a year and a half later.

A major study by the National Heart, Lung, and Blood Institute found much the same thing. Among 780 patients with chronic heart disease, half were given surgery and half treated with standard heart drugs. Five years later, the authors concluded, there was no significant difference in mortality between the two groups. The same thing was found by a group of investigators in Houston, in a study published this year in the *New England Journal of Medicine*. Clearly, this operation would seem, at best, to have a neutral effect, and given the other associated risks, it seems wiser to avoid it if at all possible.

Yet in the peculiar logic of our medical machine, that same operation—coronary bypass surgery—has become one of the "hottest" procedures on the medical charts. In 1970, only 10,000 people each year had these expensive, dangerous procedures. By 1981, there were *eleven times* as many, 110,000 each year. By 1986 the number had more than doubled again—240,000 were performed. But as those numbers rose, some others dropped: the percentage of people who survived the operation. In 1982, out of every 200 patients having four-artery bypass surgery, 194 at least came out alive. By 1985, however, that number had dropped to 192—yet surgeons performed twice as many of them each year. Simple arithmetic shows that, given so many bypasses being attempted, there are today many more deaths attributable to the operation. If these numbers seem disturbing, you're right—more operations, a lower survival rate—all for a procedure that, for many patients, may not always be necessary in the first place!

Even more staggering is their colossal price tag: Each coronary bypass costs approximately $30,000. So many people had them last year that this single operation alone accounted for $7.2 billion, almost 2 percent of the $425 billion we spent for health care in all. One would hope that the other 98 percent of our money was put to better use, but I fear that's not the case.

## Medical Orphans

Not all of the sins of our medical system are sins of commission. Many millions of Americans suffer from sins of medical omission as well. That is the case with the millions of people who suffer from what are termed "orphan diseases."

Orphans are simply rare diseases that affect fewer than twenty thousand Americans. Their rarity means several things. First, the pharmaceutical companies historically have tended to ignore them. With only, say, five thousand people afflicted with a given disease, they can't be sure that they will make enough money to justify developing a drug. Instead, they put their resources to more commonly needed, and more profitable, products. That means that, even though there may be the medical potential to create helpful, even life saving drugs, these compounds stay on the shelf, never brought to market to help people. The system makes sense for the bottom line of the drug companies, but if you or someone you love is unfortunate enough to be one of the estimated twenty million Americans suffering from an orphan disease, it is the cruelest of medical privations.

This recently got so bad that Congress stepped in. Five years ago, legislators passed a law giving financial incentives to drug manufacturers that improved their development of orphan drugs. Since then, 159 such drugs have been made available. But there are many more still needed to ease the life-destroying agonies endured by many millions of Americans.

But drugs are only half of the "orphan" problem. Because of their rarity, orphan diseases are often unrecognized by most primary-care doctors. They are the "back-of-the-textbook" diseases, rarely fully learned about and soon forgotten in a medical training system that is glutted with facts. These are the diseases, I remember from my own medical training, about which our professors said, "Look, you'll never even see a case." But even then I remember thinking, *Since they* do *exist,* some *physician has to see them.* And when we do, we as often as not have long since forgotten anything we might ever have known about them.

That means these diseases often go unrecognized and undiagnosed. "It is not unusual to hear of people being misdiagnosed for five to ten years," reports Abby Meyers, president of the National Association of Rare Disorders. "Or babies who are not diagnosed until autopsy." It has been estimated that there are as many as five thousand of these diseases. Numerically, each may afflict only a few thousand, or even a few hundred, people. But numbers aren't much comfort if you happen to be one of those people. Taken together, these orphans add up to a massive loophole of suffering and neglect in the way we do medicine.

## Ready for the Good News?

I started this chapter with the fact that something is wrong with the way we commit medicine in this country. All of the gaps in our medical safety net—the unsafe drugs, poor controls, rampant infections, unnecessary procedures—represent knowledge that our doctors don't learn in school. In the best of all worlds, young physicians would learn how to give *only safe* drugs, how *not* to infect people needlessly, and how *not* to operate unnecessarily. In short, how not to jeopardize their patients. But in the less-than-perfect world of modern medicine, those schools exist to turn out physicians who can function in the real world of insurance forms and mortgage payments, who can offer what their patients seek—high-tech, high-intensity, highly interventionist medicine.

I took the time to take you through this chapter because it is important that every person who deals with modern medicine—and that is all of us—have his or her eyes open. Only by really understanding the risks can we be intelligent, safe, and healthy medical consumers. None of us can afford to go into the health care system without knowing the truth about what we're up against.

But I promise there is good news too. By being your own advocate, really understanding how the establishment works, and *by making up yourself for what the medical machine lacks,* you can turn it to your own advantage and beat the system. That's what the second part of this book is about. Remember just because your doctor didn't learn it in medical school doesn't mean you can't learn it—now!

# 3

# Money, Medicine, and Morals

Julie G.'s ordeal began sometime after her divorce. The mother of three small children, one of whom was severely handicapped, Julie had always managed to support her family on her slim teacher's salary. Theirs was not a fancy life, she knew, but she took a warm pride in always providing her children the essentials: their comfortable, if spare home, a loving family life, the closeness of being together to support and nurture one another.

Then, one day, she returned from the family doctor with shattering news. Her doctor had detected some abnormal cell growth in her uterus. Tests confirmed the diagnosis: lethal carcinoma of her uterine wall. Her physician wasted no words. Julie's only hope, he explained, was immediate surgery. The longer she waited . . . he just let his sentence hang.

Julie knew the doctor intended his words as a reprieve, but to her, they felt like a death sentence. Surgery, she knew, meant she would not be able to start work in the new school year—and because she worked on a yearly contract, that meant no job, and no insurance. Her scant savings could not begin to cover the three thousand dollars such an operation would cost. Frantic and sick, she tried every possibility she could think of, but kept hitting brick walls. Ineligible for one program, earning too much to qualify for the next, yet always without enough money for the operation that would save her. And even if she could miraculously scrape together funds for the operation, she agonized, where would the money come from for her children to live on during her lengthy convalescence? During weeks of delay, she felt her cancer growing bigger inside her.

Desperate, she saw only one hope: Across the Atlantic, in England, she had heard, the National Health Service provided quality care free of charge. There, in a foreign land, among strangers, lay her only hope of eventually being able to see her children grow up. Anguished and frightened, she boarded a plane for London.

Within two weeks, the surgery was behind her, and after a short convalescence, Julie returned. Her doctors held out no promises, she knew, but she was grateful for whatever reprieve medical science had granted her. At best, it meant a new life; if not, at least it meant some precious time with her family, time to square things away. But as she stepped off the plane back home, Julie harbored no illusions. She knew her gift came in spite of, not because of, "the world's most advanced" medical system. Had she counted on that, she realized bitterly, she could very well be dead by now.

Few would argue that Julie was a medical victim. But what happened to her family has nothing to do with doctor-caused, iatrogenic problems. She caught no lethal germs, took no bad medicines, her physicians made no mistakes, performed no unnecessary or careless procedures. The medical professionals played their roles admirably, in strict accordance with the rules of the game. What was wrong here—very, inhumanly wrong—was those rules themselves. The fundamental problem was the assumptions that allowed this mother of three children—or any of us, for that matter—to be deprived of decent, affordable care. Julie's case exemplifies a sin of medical omission, not one of commission, but it illuminates a very basic flaw in the very cornerstone of our whole health care edifice.

For we have some basic conceptions about health care—who gets it, how, and how much—that can amount to a prescription for disease and death. They are built into the foundations of the medical monolith, and it's these rules I want to examine briefly, because they have every bit as much to do with the care you get—and what you can do about it—as the competence of your doctors, the quality of the drugs you take, or the risks in the operating theater.

There is no doubt that certain givens in our medical system can—and do—interfere with the most rational, most appropriate, and most human care. But it is equally certain that there are things each of us can do to make the system work for us, to take control of our own medical destinies.

## Blood Money

The human body's blood is red, but the life blood of our medical system is most decidedly of another hue: green, exactly the shade of money. Consider a few salient facts that, I think, put things into perspective better than the longest academic discourses ever could:

- In the first half of 1986, fees for medical-office visits rose by an average of 12 percent.
- Last year, medical costs as a whole rose 7.7 percent, exactly *seven times* the rise in general consumer prices. Although this was the largest gap between the medical economy and the overall economy in history, this trend has become a sorry fact of life in the last three decades. Between 1950 and 1977, doctors' fees rose 43 percent faster than did nonmedical care prices, reports the journal *Medical Economics*. Even worse, according to Princeton researchers, our country's health costs have climbed faster in the last five years than ever before.
- The nation's largest nonprofit hospital made a surplus of 16 percent in 1984; its for-profit counterpart had revenues of $5 billion the next year.
- More than one-sixth of all health care funds—$78 billion in one recent year—go not to doctors, not to hospitals,

and not for drugs. The money goes to process paperwork.

Such statistics can go on and on, but they all point to a clear and inescapable conclusion: Money is the driving engine behind our medical care system—and that doesn't necessarily bring the best medical care. It's not that medical capitalism cannot coexist with medical compassion, but right now there is a real question whether they do.

I recently read the annual report for America's largest hospital corporation, which boasts that its earnings per share have nearly tripled in the last five years. That is certainly good news for their stockholders, but I found myself asking if it is indeed the soundest, and most humane, way to run an institution dedicated to healing.

The answer, I fear, is no. What seems clear is that, although American medicine is awash with money—$452 billion of it this year—we aren't necessarily buying the world's best health. We have only to look abroad to see that. Take the case of Singapore: For every dollar you and your family spend on health—and it averages about $1,600 per person each year—a family in Singapore spends only $200—one-eighth as much. Yet babies born in both countries have exactly the same life expectancy. If they can get the same benefits by spending only one-eighth as much, we might all wonder just what the other seven-eighths of our health care dollars are really buying.

We see the same lesson proving true in our own nation's capital. People living in the District of Columbia spend the most each year to stay healthy, an average of $2,400 annually. Yet those same D.C. residents have a shorter life span than people living in any other state! At home and abroad, the lesson is clear: Throwing money at illness doesn't buy us health.

## Expensive Neglect: The Medical Untouchables

There is so much extra money pouring through the medical machine that at least we should be confident that everybody has access to the benefits of care. Unfortunately, in spite of the deluge of dollars, there remain many, many Americans—millions of them in fact—who never benefit from the world's richest, fattest medical monolith. Who are they?

"Many high-risk pregnant women are going without the care they should have, and infants are being exposed to permanent damage," said Robert M. Ball, commissioner of social security under three recent presidents, in recent testimony before Congress. This is so, he explained, because we have no system "guaranteeing health care for all."

This is true, too, for our seniors. "Medical schools have only one-fifth the number of teachers needed to instruct young doctors in the care of the elderly," says Dr. T. Franklin Williams, director of the National Institute for Aging.

*More than one in five* lower- and fixed-income people cannot afford vital blood pressure medication their doctor has prescribed, reports the *American Journal of Public Health.*

A black child born within five miles of Washington, D.C., has less chance of living to celebrate his first birthday than a similar child born in many Third World countries, among them Jamaica, Trinidad, and Tobago, says the Children's Defense Fund.

Seniors, babies, pregnant women, poor people—all are being increasingly dealt out of the world's richest health care system. One can hardly pick up a newspaper or magazine today without reading about some way in which our medical values have been skewed and distorted due to economic pressures.

There is no better example than what happened to one of my recent patients. Mrs. M., a middle-aged woman, came in to see me in great distress. She suffered from a panoply of obviously allergic symptoms: severe skin rashes, hives, swelling, and crippling joint pain. I suggested a standard blood test, called a RAST test, to isolate the substances that were causing her problems. Her eyes began to fill with tears: "But doctor, before I came here, I went to an allergist in my town, and he said the same thing. But then he told me the test costs four hundred dollars, and I . . . well, I can't afford it," her voice quavered. "So he said he could draw the blood, freeze it, and then run the test when I had the money." My jaw dropped. That this woman, in obvious pain, with an entirely preventable problem, was being frankly denied an essential test until she could cough up four hundred dollars set my head spinning. Thank heaven, most doctors would never think of such an arrangement, and I found it hard to believe hers had. Shaking my head, I sent her for her test right then and there.

Not a week later the point was brought home to me again. I picked up a copy of *The New York Times* and read an article reporting that all the obstetricians serving a community of seventy thousand in Rhode Island had begun turning away low-income pregnant women. They could not provide prenatal care, they said, because Medicaid does not pay them enough to keep their doors open.

The fact is those physicians are fighting an uphill battle: When you count their costs of insurance and the slim fee paid by Medicaid, they actually *lose money* each time they see a patient. Under such a fundamentally flawed system, it is no surprise that even the most dedicated and well-intentioned of physicians find themselves adopting a mercenary outlook.

Above that article, on the same page, another article stated that an effort to limit the advertising of cigarettes had met with yet another defeat. At issue was not whether the practice was life-endangering—everybody agreed it was—but whether it was permissible to interfere in the tobacco companies' "right to advertise."

I could not help think, as I laid down the paper, that the juxtaposition of these two reports put in stark relief just how far we have twisted our medical values in the name of profit. It is shameful that the "world's best" medical system can neither deliver basic prenatal care to poor women nor take an affirmative stand on a proven killer that costs thousands of lives each year.

Even the pages of our professional medical journals reflect the fact that our healing priorities have been gravely affected by the distortions of profit-motive medicine. The *New England Journal of Medicine* reports that a recent study from Northwestern University examined patients "dumped" at a public hospital from other hospitals in the Chicago area. Of these, 89 percent were black or Hispanic, and 81 percent had no job. The hospitals quite baldly listed the reasons for most of those transfers as "inadequate medical insurance." Of course, it would be one thing if those patients were merely being transferred to receive similar or better care. But the authors' conclusions suggested something much more chilling: "Patients are transferred predominantly for economic reasons, in spite of the fact that many of them are in an unstable condition," they wrote. More alarming, these researchers found that such "dumped" patients died more than twice as often as other patients. One can't help wondering how many of those people would be alive today if hospitals looked more at the medical chart and less at the ledger book.

## Buried in the Insurance Avalanche

I recently attended a symposium where I was asked to select the single most significant medical development in the last thirty years. I didn't pick a CT scanner or a heart transplant. My answer wasn't some great new drug or computer-enhanced procedure. I think that the biggest medical change in my lifetime is no thicker than a single sheet of paper. In fact, it is a sheet of paper—the insurance form.

Actually, it isn't the paper itself that is significant but the immense for-profit bureaucracy that lurks behind it. Together, they have transformed the face of American health more than any other tool, drug, or procedure. And as anyone knows who has been caught in their unholy bureaucracy—and that means doctors, every bit as much as patients—that change is definitely a mixed blessing.

For the first time in history, there is a strange new player in the medical drama. No longer is healing a private matter among doctor, patient, and family. Today, some of the most powerful players in the health care system are those concerned not with health but with money. Theirs is a bottom-line approach to health. Ensuring accessible, high-quality care is not their main goal; generating dividends is. That should make all of us more than a bit concerned.

## Slicing the Payment Pie

Thirty-five years ago—when many of the doctors now in practice were just starting their medical careers—the medical relationship involved only doctors, patients, and their families. In those days, you did what you thought best for the patient, and nobody looked over your shoulder. Back then, the medical-payment pie looked like the graph on page 50.

As you can see, most of the cost was paid by people themselves. But since then, inch by inch, the insurance payers have taken over a larger and larger role in our way of healing, so that today, the pie graph looks like that on page 51.

In other words, people pay just about half the percentage of their medical bills they once did, government pays about twice as much, and private insurance pays more than three times as much.

On the face of it, that seems like a relief for all of us

## Percentage of Medical Bills in 1950 Paid by . . .

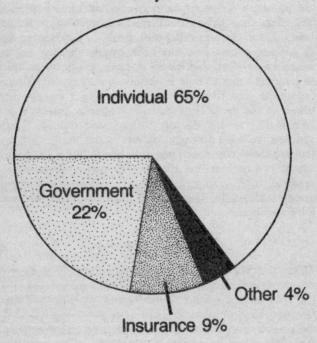

Individual 65%

Government 22%

Insurance 9%

Other 4%

and our families. But, at a much more insidious level, it has meant the explosive growth of a huge, unwieldy health breaucracy. That has led to figures that would have seemed pure, nonsensical fantasy just a few years ago. That we spend more than one-sixth of all health care funds on paperwork and administrative costs is, in a word, ludicrous. In the most recent year for which we have records, experts put this cost at a staggering $78 billion. Tens of billions of dollars that don't buy a single operating room, pay for a single nurse's time, or purchase a single

# Percentage of Medical Bills in 1985 Paid by . . .

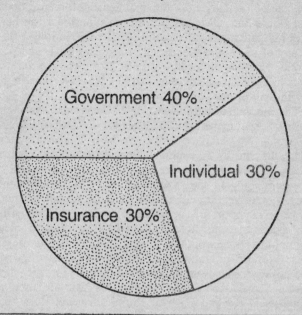

pill, but merely push around the paper that our system thrives on.

In our own lives, every one of us has experienced the deluge of paperwork that accompanies even the most minor of medical visits. Forms in triplicate, insurance cards, preadmission certifications, receipts, canceled checks, reimbursement records, deductible vouchers—the list is endless. What patients see is actually only the tiniest tip of a huge iceberg of paper and procedures.

## Who's in Charge Here?

Today, with doctors, hospitals, administrators, insurance companies, actuaries, health maintenance organizations, and Uncle Sam all in the act, the relationship I can have with my patients is fundamentally altered. No longer do I or any of my colleagues simply diagnose, treat, and prescribe. Now we also administrate. And there are times it feels like we have been relegated to a bit-player role in the health care of our patients.

The most disturbing aspect of the Insurance Avalanche is that it has opened the medical doors to whole legions of people who aren't doctors. We have created a system of health care by bureaucrats. Because insurance companies pay the bills, they are able to shift the direction of new technologies and treatments. Only those treatments they reimburse for will flourish and be accepted; those they don't support are consigned to medical oblivion. That has meant that our most innovative, prevention-oriented, commonsense approaches—things such as regular physicals, exercise programs, and nutritional counseling—are not covered. What are covered are the very drastic, dangerous, costly procedures—techniques that are used as stopgaps at the end stage of chronic diseases. In a very real way, the insurers' policies have become the engines driving a counterproductive and health-destroying system of care.

## The Great Insurance Bailout

What is even more galling is that now the insurers are madly trying to scramble out of their end of the bargain. For two decades, insurance largely insulated people from what medical care really costs. That helped send costs skyrocketing through the roof. But now that the costs are so high, insurers want to be exempt from paying for whole classes of illnesses.

First they hit us with what they termed "preexisting

conditions"—in practice, that meant anything that was wrong with you that they could conceivably use to deny you payment. I recently saw a patient who had allergic problems as a child twenty years ago, but who has been healthy, productive (and, I might add, paying premiums) since then. When he came to my office with a breathing problem, his insurance company tried to withhold payment, claiming that it was a long-standing allergic condition—in spite of the fact that he had never had these symptoms before and hadn't manifested any severe allergic symptoms for almost a quarter of a century! Despairing, he asked me, "What have I been paying for all these years if the first time I really need it, they tell me I'm ineligible?"

Even more disturbing, now insurers want to bail out from having to cover specific expensive diseases. The most blatant example is AIDS, where they are trying to require blood tests in order to get insured. In other words, only if they can be fairly sure you won't get the disease will they agree to insure you for it. That may be a great cost-cutting deal for them, but it runs against the basic premise of insurance—spreading risk—and it is grossly unfair for the rest of us.

AIDS is just the beginning. Today, in research laboratories throughout the world, scientists are discovering blood-test markers for many chronic, hereditary diseases, including Alzheimer's disease, muscular dystrophy, cystic fibrosis, and hemophilia. With each new test, insurers will try to add them to the list of disqualifying screens—reducing their economic risk while increasing our health risk. After all, if they can exclude AIDS, why not cancer and heart disease? As they expand such programs, it means that more and more of us risk becoming "insurance untouchables," excluded from coverage because blood tests suggest we might, of all things, actually get sick and file a claim!

These insurance giants would like nothing better than to insure only the healthiest people and exclude the rest of us. It is the same backward thinking that leads them to cover surgery but not the life-style education that could reduce the need for surgery. But for the rest of us, it is a dangerous and destructive trend. After all, these companies are already making huge profits with the system as it is now. The last thing we need is a development that increases their revenues while denying people protection. The whole idea of insurance, recall, is that you spread the risk, not eliminate it!

Besides, I assure you, if they are allowed to bail out of covering anybody who is likely to get sick, and so slash their own risk, we won't see them lower their insurance rates. They will pass the savings along not to their members but to their stockholders. We must never forget that these companies exist to create not health, but wealth—because certainly they never forget it.

## The Money-Medicine Muddle

Clearly, more and more medical decisions are being made on the basis of judgments that are far from being purely therapeutic. Equally clearly, in my view, the more money meddles in medicine, the more it muddles medicine. It seems that everywhere I turn I see examples of the way economics have skewed our medical values and practices.

For example, it would seem obvious that doctors who do the same thing should charge the same thing. Yet a recent survey by the attorney general of Maryland tells a very different story. Doctors' fees for the exact same procedure varied by as much as 333 percent from one physician to the next. The surveyors found that price differences don't depend on quality of care, or speed of service, or degree of the physician's time or training. Instead, it seems that younger physicians, with loans to pay off and expensive offices to set up, tend to charge higher fees. Does it make sense that your bill should depend not on what is wrong or what is done but on your doctor's bank balance? No—it's a product of the money-medicine muddle.

A study in Montreal reported a similar trend. When Canada began a national health care plan, physicians radically altered what they did with their patients. Most significantly, there was an abrupt decline in those procedures and services that take more of a doctor's time and a "redirecting of services to better paying activities."

A similar point echoes in a fascinating study from Colorado. There it was found that when the government reduced how much physicians could charge under Medicare by 10 percent, the kind of medicine they practiced changed noticeably. Surgical procedures rose 1.4 percent, physicians reported a 6 percent increase in complex procedures, and they ordered 5 percent more lab tests. Taken together, the increase totaled 12.4 percent—handsomely making up for the 10 percent reduction in Medicare payments.

What we are seeing is the clear result of medicine-by-bureaucracy. For it is a truism that the more our medicine is steered by administrators and cost accountants, and the less doctors are free to practice the best kind of doctoring they know how to, the easier it is for decisions to drift from the purely medical to the more unabashedly economic. It is a very fundamental—and a very flawed—way of healing.

That is not good news for any of us. Not long ago, a congressional committee reported a story from a New Jersey hospital. It seems a hospital administrator suggested that one physician rethink his practice of rarely counseling pregnant patients to undergo caesarean sections. The reason? The state's diagnosis-based payment system rates this riskier, more traumatic procedure higher than nonsurgical means of childbirth—so the hospital makes more money doing it. The report didn't state what the physician's response was, nor what has happened to his pregnant patients since then.

I find this incident particularly disturbing, because this same system of diagnosis-related payments, which was then being tested in New Jersey, is now being applied in all fifty states. That can only mean that such cases, and the pressure to make medical decisions with an eye to the bottom line instead of the patients' welfare, will increase. Happily, this physician made the only right moral decision, by refusing to change his practices and endanger his patients. But under this new system, how many more physicians this year will be pressured to cut corners?

## Cancer Cash and Carry

Just recently, a colleague of mine, a cancer specialist, told me about a new cancer care center in Tennessee. They offer state-of-the-art treatments with a new anticancer tool called monoclonal antibiodies. But what is different about this clinic is that it requires its patients to pay for their own research. The highly experimental treatments they offer are not yet proven or available for use in general hospitals. Such cutting-edge treatments are usually only available in major research centers, with strict controls, funded by government or industry grants. But instead, this clinic charges the guinea-pig patients themselves—often up to thirty-five thousand dollars for their two-week course of treatments. That means, of course, that only those who can afford such a monumental price tag will be treated. It is, in its simplest terms, cancer care where only the wealthy need apply.

The defenders of such profit-motive medicine claim they provide treatments not available elsewhere. As to the inequity of it, they seem to shrug it off, as though of course people should expect to pay top dollar for specialized treatment. Perhaps such a clinic is an inevitable next step in the trend to privatized health care. But I think we must ask if it is not instead a symptom of a system breaking down, of the triumph of economic factors over humanitarian judgment. We should all take a long, hard look at whether any of us benefit when we create a system of "checkbook health care."

I wish I could say these examples are uncommon, but they really are not. I doubt there is a practicing physician in this country who could not add his or her own anecdotes about the medicine-money muddle. I guarantee you that if you were to have a chat with your own family practitioner, you would hear more of the same. It's not your doctor's fault. You may be lucky enough to have a doctor who is caring, responsible, and devoted, but, like all of us, that doctor is caught in a system not of his own making.

As a physician, I seem to see this unfortunate trend worsen every day. Far too often, I know that all these examples boil down to one fundamentally disturbing trend: Decisions that should be medical, personal judgments between doctor and patient are being made by phalanxes of cost accountants, administrators, and bureaucrats. As one internist recently put it, "The Hippocratic oath of *'primum non nocere'* is often translated as 'above all, do no harm.' Now it's being replaced by *'primum non expendere'*—'above all, do not spend.' "

## Prevention: The Neglected Stepchild

Of all the ways in which money muddles medicine, there is none so glaring as our wholesale neglect of preventive strategies for health. Our current medical-payment system works as a clear incentive to be sick and gives us no reinforcement whatsoever for staying well. One could not have designed a more efficient system to keep America unhealthy. Our insurers cover radical open-heart surgery, invasive diagnostic tests, and dangerous radiation therapy, yet refuse reimbursement for basic programs of fitness, exercise, and life-style and nutrition counseling, which could help make such radical procedures largely obsolete.

I can recall, during my medical school training, attending a day-long seminar on cancer. We heard about drugs and surgeries, laser treatments, radiation, and chemotherapy—but not one of the learned doctors spoke about the preventive steps that could help our patients avoid cancer in the first place. Until recently, that was the state of the art. If you are one of those whose doctor has actually taken the time to counsel you about the many preventive steps you can take for such killers as cancer, heart disease, high blood pressure, and stroke, you should consider yourself lucky—and give your physician a nod of thanks. For those are the exceptional physicians, and you are lucky to have one.

Still, for far too many, preventive medicine remains a *terra incognita* on the medical map. It seems strange it should be that way. After all, you hardly need an advanced degree to recognize that it makes little sense to haul people into our hospitals, dose them with powerful drugs, and subject them to disfiguring, dangerous therapies when, instead, we could help them to lead the kinds of lives that make such radical steps unnecessary.

The Public Health Research Group in Washington, D.C., estimates that we spend about $100 billion each year on medical care for entirely preventable illnesses. As staggering a sum as that is, other experts place the true cost even higher. At a recent Senate hearing, Joseph Califano, former secretary of Health, Education and Welfare, estimated that fully *two-thirds* of all disease and premature death is preventable. Following these calculations, we spend some $250 billion each year on conditions that need not exist.

Today, in 1988, we have more knowledge than we ever had before about the ways in which people can prevent illness and ensure a long and healthy life. We have developed an armamentarium of preventive principles that work, and work well. Prevention holds significant promise for problems as diverse as cancer, heart and blood-vessel disease, stroke, immune disorders, and a huge range of chronic, debilitating diseases from pernicious anemia to osteoporosis.

Experts estimate that simply by taking advantage of the preventive measures we now know about—such staples as proper exercise, improved diet, stress reduction, not smoking, early medical screening, and reducing exposure to dangerous chemicals—we could reduce by fully two-thirds our incidence of serious illness.

In some areas, to be sure, we have already started seeing great prevention payoffs. Most dramatic is that having to do with heart-attack death. Three out of ten people are alive today who would have died from coronary attacks twenty years ago. Epidemiologists attribute the difference directly to preventive life-style measures. That is the best payoff possible: human lives saved.

But in other areas, the medical monolith has been slow to pick up on this new way of viewing health. Until quite recently, and still today in many sections of the country, strong preventive measures still play only a minor supporting role in our medical drama. Center stage is still occupied by our antiquated, illness-centered vision of healing. We still define medical care as "fixing what's wrong." Viewing health care that way is like going to a symphony where the musicians do nothing but tune up and the crescendo never comes. The promise of true preventive health care is so much broader than that. It has ramifications for our health, our vitality, our ability to fight off disease and lead full, rich, energetic lives.

## What Would Hippocrates Say?

To be sure, we have seen some glimmers of a new, fresh way of viewing preventive medicine. One comes from my own alma mater, Tufts Medical School. For the first time, in May of 1986, Tufts graduates broke tradition by not taking the Hippocratic Oath. Instead, they swore allegiance to a new vision of preventive medicine. That oath read, in part, "I will prevent disease whenever I can, for prevention is preferable to cure." The new oath also emphasized the healing power of a close, mutual doctor-patient relationship: "I will remember that there is art to medicine as well as science, and that warmth, sympathy, and understanding may outweigh the surgeon's knife or the chemist's drug." I can't help but think that we are finally coming back around to medical truths that Hippocrates, the first doctor, knew long ago.

Unfortunately, such enlightenment remains the too-rare exception to the medical rule. For the most part, our medical system continues to practice "reactive medicine," groaning and creaking along under the weight of its profound limitations. As a result, one in four Americans are still overweight, despite all we know about the links between overweight and heart attack, coronary artery disease, diabetes, cancer, and stroke. The most recent figures from the secretary of Health and Human Services show that fewer than one American in five exercises strenuously and often enough to derive aerobic benefit to reduce heart attack risk.

Research cardiologists admit that while some of the message has gotten through to what used to be the highest-risk group—middle-aged, male executives—it has spread less well among ordinary working people. What that suggests is that those with the most access to sources of information outside the health care system have begun to get the message, but that others haven't caught up yet. When it comes to preventive health care, perhaps the sorriest statistic of all is the fact that a staggering fifty-three million Americans still haven't gotten the message about tobacco, and continue to smoke.

There is no doubt that we still lumber along with a system where far too much medicine happens in emergency rooms, and not enough in classrooms. Because of that, about one million people will die of heart disease this year alone. Our medical system has to get the message across, to patients and practitioners alike, that it is wiser for doctors to spend an hour explaining and teaching in their offices now than to spend two weeks visiting their patients in the hospital five years from now.

Perhaps not surprisingly, it is our businesses, which foot such a large share of our medical bills, that have been among the first to see the light about prevention. Across the country, in test programs from New York to Los Angeles, studies show that people who work in corporations, unions, schools, and organizations with preventive health programs have fewer sick days, reduced disability claims, and lower doctor bills than their fellows who don't take preventive measures. Preventive health programs also lower the rates of absenteeism, job turnover, and job fatigue, and increase overall health.

Unfortunately, I wish I could say that our government has been as quick to get the message, but they haven't. When it comes to prevention, they have not done even a tiny fraction of what they should to encourage the health of our people. Today, our nation spends less than 1 percent of the health care budget on preventive measures. History will record a cruel irony that during the same years when we have learned just how dramatically prevention can save lives, we have watched our budgets for such programs dwindle. In the last seven years, funds for preventive health programs have dropped drastically—to the tune of $217 million.

You may notice that throughout this last section, I have talked about prevention largely in terms of dollars and cents. That makes it easier to quantify, and easier to be objective. But every day I practice medicine it is not the economics I see but the very human side of this equation. That is much harder for me to accept.

It is wrenching to see my waiting room filled with people whose lives have been shattered by needless suffering, debility, and death, people whose medical trials could have been avoided if only someone had taken the time to inform and educate them about how they could live their lives differently—before it is too late. These people are the true victims of our old-fashioned, illness-based medicine, and they are the ones who have the most to gain by our over-hauling the medical machine. The rest of this book is dedicated to those people, to the doctors who are trying to help them, and to all of us who want to take control over our health.

# 4

# Are You "Doctor-Wise"?

When her husband, Bob, went into the hospital for tests, Vivian G. didn't know what to think. Sixty-two years old, he had been diagnosed with Parkinson's disease several months ago, but his symptoms had recently gotten much worse. Bob had already been through so much: two years ago, open-heart surgery, then a serious case of acquired hepatitis from a contaminated blood transfusion. Since then, she thought, he had never been quite right. He was tired all the time, irritable and spiritless. No more did she hear his stirring Irish tenor filling the house with "Danny Boy." Now he just sat in his armchair and slept.

Their doctor had little hope to offer. "Your husband has been through a lot," he explained. "He received so many blood transfusions, well, we never know what could be down the line for him. We know the blood gave him hepatitis, but, well, there could be other contaminants . . ." Instantly, her mind spun as she read between the lines. The doctor didn't come out and say it, but she knew he was suggesting her husband might have AIDS. Of course, that explained Bob's tiredness and fatigue, the gradual withering away of the vital man who had been her husband. "He may want to be tested," the doctor finished. "It's your decision."

Vivian felt herself going numb. In the day it took her to reach her twenty-five-year-old daughter, Emily, she felt like she was in a terrible, cold vacuum. When she finally reached her daughter, Vivian felt herself begin to come apart. Shaking, choking out the words, she relayed the doctor's message.

"She assumed the worst, that Dad definitely had AIDS and that was that," recalls Emily. Because her mother had been so shaken, she didn't seem to understand very clearly what the doctor had said, so Emily called him herself. But that second conversation went very differently.

No, the doctor didn't think he had AIDS. In fact, the odds were against it, he said. No, he didn't think her father's symptoms were necessarily anything more than complications of his Parkinson's. No, her father had not been tested for AIDS. In fact, he wouldn't recommend that he take the blood test, because the psychological trauma alone could make him worse, and it wouldn't prove anything. And no, he didn't have any reason to suspect that there necessarily had been other blood contaminants. "Look," he clarified, "I just wanted someone in the family to be aware, so you'd know there is a decision you could make if you want to. It's up to you." As Emily got off the phone, she was crying, too—but hers were tears of relief.

The terror and stress of what happened to Emily's family was entirely avoidable. Emily and her mother had been put on psychological red alert, going through agony simply because of a sorry miscommunication. When Emily told me the story some weeks later, it reaffirmed something I had long observed among my patients: that some people just know how to deal with doctors, and the whole medical system, more effectively than others do, and they do better in our medical system.

I recall reading an article stating that one reason patients may not follow their physician's recommendations is that they feel they never really got the chance to explain to their doctor what is wrong with them. According to the researcher at the University of North Carolina, patients may explain only a little bit of their complaint before the doctor prematurely terminates the exam and prescribes something. Feeling unheard, and less than supremely confident, such people may not comply with their doctor's counsel. After all, they may figure, what does he know— he didn't even hear what I had to say! Again, it's a typical case of doctor-patient communication actually blocking the best care.

Contrast that with someone like Emily, who is "doctor-wise." Because of the attitude she took toward her father's care—questioning, assertive, and confident—she was able to interact with their doctor in a way her mother simply could not. Where her mother panicked, deferred to the physician, and was left to draw her own, very frightening conclusions, Emily had a different style. She pinned the doctor down on *exactly* what he meant, probed for details, confronted him with questions, and listened until she was sure she understood. Obviously, had Emily been on the phone in the first place, both she and her mother, and even their doctor, could have avoided needless stress, sorrow, and worry.

Emily knows that becoming "doctor-wise" is an invaluable skill in our current medical system. The truth is, it is up to all of us to look out for ourselves and the welfare of those we love, because too often the system doesn't do it for us. If you are lucky, your doctor may have gone over the basics of good nutrition and healthy exercise with you, but I doubt very much that you have ever gotten any guidance about how to make yourself a more effective consumer in our medical marketplace.

Because you have read this far, I hope that that has begun to change. I expect that you have already begun to get past a major hurdle: medical passivity. You may have opened this book believing the comforting doctrine that doctors are all-knowing. Like most people, you have been brought up to think that you get the best medical care when you place yourself lock, stock, and barrel into your physician's hands. I hope these last chapters have helped change your attitude on that score.

The goal of this chapter is to talk about how all of us can improve our skills for coping with medical problems, events, and decisions. I guarantee you, in a few pages you will already start to feel more confident and knowledgeable—in short, more "doctor-wise."

## Cooperation: The Best RX of All

It is a fact of modern medical care that the best care comes when patients and their physicians work as a team. You may think of your physician as the one with all the expertise—but the reality is that each side brings an expertise to making your health all it can be.

When I step into an examining room with a patient, I know that I am there to be part of a team. On my side, I offer my specialized knowledge, schooling, and experience; on yours, you bring your judgment, your personal values, and your own sense of what works and what doesn't—for you. Both are equally important. That's why the second half of this book's title is so important—after all, what counts is not just your doctor's training—what they did or didn't learn in medical school—but what *you* can do about it. And *doing*, in this case, means teamwork.

## Welcome to Your Health Care Team!

Study after study shows that those people who take a more active role in their own health care—who see themselves as more in control, making more decisions about their own care—do better on every available measure of health. A sampling of the literature reveals a clear and provocative pattern:

- Researchers at the Veterans Administration Hospital in Houston compared two groups of men recovering from major kidney operations. They found that men who accepted responsibility and assumed a role in understanding and clarifying their surgeon's explanations and who deliberated on their doctors' recommendations instead of just blindly accepting them recovered faster and better from surgery. The common link, say the researchers, is that the healthier men were active participants, not passive recipients of their medical care.

- Dr. Judith Rodin, a researcher at Yale University, reports that nursing-home patients who were encouraged to make more of their own choices and feel more in control got more active, felt better, and showed greater overall health improvements than those who were encouraged to wait passively while the hospital staff filled their needs. Even more suggestive, reported the researchers, was that the "in control" group actually had a lower death rate than the passive group! Her paper also cites several studies showing that people who "feel helpless take longer to recover from illness or are more likely to die from serious illness."

- Psychiatrists examined a group of women with irregular Pap smears, who were at risk for developing cancer. They found that those women who felt helpless and out of control were much more likely to actually develop cancers than those who felt they were in command of their health.

- Physicians have shown that patients who have more information and a sense of participating in surgical procedures experience less pain, need less medication, and heal faster from surgery than those who feel like passive recipients of their doctors' procedures.

What is clear, from these studies and scores of others, is that all of us do better, physically, psychologically, and even physiologically, when we take an active, involved, role in our own process of getting better—the exact opposite of "handing it over to the experts and hoping for the best."

## Trust: The Vital Ingredient

I am not saying your shouldn't trust your own physician. Of course you should. He or she can be your most potent ally both in keeping you healthy and in getting you better when you're not. I very much hope that you are one of the many people who has a family doctor you trust completely, whose advice has proven itself over the years, and who knows your special needs and the factors that make you unique. You can consider yourself lucky to be taking advantage of the American healing system at its best.

But for all of us there are times and situations when the ideal of a close, long-term health care partnership is not met. There may be times when your personal doctor sends you to a specialist who doesn't know you so well, who doesn't have the benefit of years of history working with you and your family. Or you may find yourself in situations where you must deal with a whole team of doctors, each working in his or her own specialty and not aware of the larger picture of you and your family's health.

Or you may be one of the millions of Americans who belong to a health maintenance organization (HMO) or group health plan. Often that means you won't see the same doctor each time you go to the clinic, and the person treating you may have little personal experience with you, your family, or your body's patterns.

For all of us, some medical happenstance is unavoidable. You may find yourself needing care far from home, while on a vacation or a business trip, when your doctor's reassuring presence is far away. Or, like many Americans, you may be planning a move or have recently relocated to a new community where you don't yet have a relationship with a physician.

In short, all of us need to know how to take an active role in our own care. We need to know when and how to stand up for ourselves so that we don't get lost in the medical shuffle. Usually, those who have learned this lesson have done so only by experience—the bitter trial of having something go wrong in the ministrations of the medical machine.

Well, the good news is that it doesn't have to be that way. Each of us can learn some basic rules ahead of time, *before* you or your family need to, so that we won't become the kind of statistics we have already discussed.

## Do Your Doctor a Favor: Get Involved

One other word about teamwork: You may have a comfortable, secure relationship with your practitioner and feel just a bit reluctant to rock the boat and start asserting yourself more in the medical process. Don't be. Believe me, if you have a responsible physician, he or she will welcome the "new you." You will actually be doing your physician a favor.

I doubt that patients always appreciate just how much we doctors *want* them to take a stronger, more active role. Despite all the public relations about doctors being invulnerable and powerful, the fact is that all but the most megalomaniacal of us prefer it when our patients work with us. Think about it—isn't that the reason that her physician telephoned Vivian in the story above—to ask for the family's support and counsel? He knew there was an important decision to be made and did not feel comfortable making it alone. In that conversation he was actually seeking out his patients' guidance—a fact that Emily recognized and was able to provide.

The same lesson was brought home to me one day during my surgical residency as I left the operating room with an orthopedic surgeon after a particularly grueling surgery. He had just spent nine hours repairing the spinal column of a massively obese man, whose vertebrae had collapsed under the stress of the extra hundred-plus pounds he was carrying. The exhausted surgeon turned to me: "What we just did in there never should have happened. I told him seven months ago he could be in trouble if he didn't lose weight." I could see he was trying to control his frustration: "Sometimes it feels like they are working just as hard as they can to defeat us." I recall thinking that that entire risky operation, and my teacher's frustration, could have been avoided by a closer, more cooperative relationship between doctor and patient—and it would have done them both good.

So if you want to know a doctor's secret, here it is: Our favorite patients are those who help us by helping themselves, taking an active, involved interest in their health. After all, if I know you are taking an active interest in having the best health you can, it makes it a lot easier for me to feel the same way.

## Six Tips to Better Health

### 1. There's No Such Thing as a Dumb Question!

*"There is nothing so complex
that it cannot be explained simply."*
—Albert Einstein

Dr. Einstein was not a medical doctor, but I wish that more physicians and patients would take this bit of his wisdom to heart. The fact is, true teamwork medicine requires that you understand as much as possible about what is happening, what is wrong, and *exactly* what you can and can't do to make things better. That brings me to my first "tip": Ask questions—and keep doing so until you understand.

For some reason, too much of our medical care has grown up around the idea that there is something wrong with being informed and asking questions. But the truth is, there is nothing wrong with asking questions, and there are very few medical conditions that can't be explained in terms you can understand.

Too often people feel that they are wasting their physicians' valuable time by asking even basic questions or requesting even a simple clarification of something they didn't quite understand. They feel that medicine is so inestimably complicated—with all those long Latinate names for things—that they couldn't possibly understand.

Nonsense. Nothing could be further from the truth. Of course you can understand. (After all, your doctor learned these facts, so you can, too!) The modern medical reality, given our move toward outpatient, at-home, and preventive medical treatment, requires more than ever that all of us be engaged in and understand what is going on. To do that, we have to feel free to ask questions, and ask them again, until we feel confident and well informed. The best physicians don't view this as an unwelcome intrusion on their time or expertise. They see it as a necessary step to creating healthier, more involved patients.

If you feel tongue-tied and embarrassed each time you want to ask your doctor a question, I suggest you answer this quick checklist:

- Does your doctor seem impatient or hurried when you start discussing your questions?
- Do you try to abbreviate or rush through your questions so that you won't keep the doctor waiting when he or she has so many other people to see?
- Are your questions met with vague, long-winded, or evasive answers?
- Do you find yourself unable to explain to friends and family what your doctor really told you?
- Do you find yourself relieved to be able to turn to nurses, nurses' aides, or orderlies to explain things to you?

If you answered yes to more than two of these, I suggest you examine whether you feel you are really getting the kind of information you want from your physician. Your response to these questions may be a tip-off that you are being encouraged in subtle—and not-so-subtle—ways to "sit back and keep quiet." I do not believe that that is the basis for safe and sound long-term medical teamwork.

## 2. Can They Pass the Interview?

A second tip that helps some patients is to approach their physicians in the same time-tested way they would approach anyone they have to work closely with, from a secretary to a baby-sitter: Interview them.

One young couple I know, call them Bill and Karen, used this technique when Karen was pregnant with their first child. "We sat down with three different obstetricians and talked about their philosophy, what we were looking for, what we did and did not feel comfortable with," recalls Karen. The idea is not so much to disqualify prospective doctors but to get an idea of which practitioner has the mix of personal style, communications skills, and a philosophy of medical practice that you feel most comfortable with.

For Karen and Bill, it was an important decision. They knew they didn't want a caesarean birth, but rather a more natural birthing experience. They felt they needed a doctor who knew how to handle any birth complications, but who would not steer them into needlessly invasive procedures or toxic drugs. After two long interviews, they found exactly the doctor they liked: a young, progressive physician in their neighborhood. Eight months later Karen gave birth to a rousingly healthy baby boy—exactly as she and Bill had always wanted it. Looking back, they would have had it no other way. "Sure, it was inconvenient, and a bit expensive, to settle on the right person," Karen admits. "But there wasn't one moment in the whole pregnancy when we didn't feel total confidence in our medical advice. And now we know we have a family doctor for the baby for the next ten years. That confidence is worth a lot."

I doubt you are used to the idea of interviewing your doctor, but some people find that it is exactly the right way to start your health care relationships off on the right footing: saying that you plan to take an active, responsible role in your health and that you seek a physician who can respect you and work with that.

### 3. Stand Up for Yourself

My third principle for being a better medical consumer is the most important of all. Once you've found the doctor you like, work to develop your own style of medical assertiveness. By this, I don't mean you have to be bossy, demanding, or unrealistic in your expectations. That won't help you, your health, or the professionals who are trying to assist you. But I do mean that you should be able to stick up for what you want, and walk away feeling that your questions have been answered and your concerns addressed.

The easiest way to do that is to keep reminding yourself of a few basic facts. *You* are the lead character in your own health. It is you who are at the same time the subject of interest, the one with the most to gain and lose, and the one paying the bills. You have a right to expect satisfaction.

But how can you translate this into real-world behavior? Some people find it helpful to hone their skills so that they can get more satisfaction from their care providers. You might actually rehearse some possible replies you can make during your annual physical: "Why, no, doctor, I don't understand that part very well. Can you please explain that last part again?" Or: "Well, what are you really telling me that I can expect next?" Or: "I'd appreciate it if you could list my options for me." Sometimes, assertiveness means calling in the help you need: "Excuse me, doctor, but I think it would help me to have my fiancé here for this discussion, so I'd like to wait until he arrives."

You may not be used to dealing with your doctor this way but once you get used to it, you'll wonder how you ever did anything else. Remember, the physician sitting opposite you in the white lab coat or the surgical greens is just another person. He or she understands fear and confusion and the need to be treated with respect. The more you take charge of your own health, the more likely it is that your physician will appreciate it and respond favorably. If he or she doesn't, you should realize that that is a limitation of that doctor's own personal style of practice. You may want to rethink whether this is the kind of health care partnership you really want.

## 4. Two Heads Are Better Than One

My fourth counsel may sound familiar, but it's amazing how few people truly follow it. In medicine, as in most things, two heads *are definitely* better than one. Yet in spite of all that has been written about the necessity of obtaining a second opinion, too many people still seem to have trouble believing this simple health care truth. In some fashion, people still feel that their doctors will view it as disloyal or untrusting. Dr. Eugene McCarthy, director of the Health Benefits Research Center of New York Hospital, has estimated that "between one-half and two-thirds" of patients who do visit another doctor don't want their primary physician to know that they are getting a second opinion.

That seems strange to me. After all, if a physician is confident of the diagnosis, he or she should welcome confirmation. If not, you as a patient deserve to know that fact. Getting a second opinion is an entirely reasonable, sane way you can begin to take control of your own health and well-being. When you consider the medical, human, and financial costs that can accompany hospitalizations and medical and surgical procedures, it is quite clear that none of us should subject ourself to such risks without some confirmation that it is necessary and prudent.

The health statisticians have understood this for a long time. They have estimated that a nationwide program of mandatory second opinions can save up to eight dollars for every health care dollar we spend, money that would otherwise be spent on needless procedures, useless surgery, and dangerous drugs. Studies reported by the Senate Committee on Aging show that when second opinions become the rule rather than the exception, overall surgical rates drop by almost half—and certain procedures drop by as much as 60 percent. In Senate testimony, Dr. Richard Kusserow, inspector general of Health and Human Services, estimates that our nation would save ninety million dollars on Medicare alone if people always got second opinions.

While the statisticians may concern themselves with the economic bottom line, most of us have a much more immediate real-world concern: We want to avoid needless pain, suffering, and disability for us and those around us. What better reason to insist on a two-heads-are-better-than-one approach, before you subject yourself to the medical machine?

## 5. Know Your Insurance

My fifth suggestion is not about doctors at all. It concerns that new, very powerful player on the health care scene: the insurers and so-called "third-party" payers. I have talked about some of the changes these have brought for physicians, but you should also know about the changes they mean for you, every time you set foot in a doctor's office, HMO clinic, or hospital. Because in a very profound way, those changes can spell the difference between excellent, adequate, and substandard care.

All of it boils down to a simple rule: Know your coverage. Too many people go along happily assuming that they will be well covered in case of medical mishap—only to find, when the time comes and they or a loved one are carried off in an ambulance, that they have become the victims of a small-print nightmare of exclusions, waivers, and limitations.

A young patient of mine named Noah W. recently found this out the hard way. Through his regular internist, Noah was admitted to the hospital for an elective procedure. His preparation, surgery, and postoperative care went flawlessly—until the bills started coming in. For some reason, his insurance company was only paying half the invoice amount. The reason? It turned out there was a new and little-publicized provision in his policy that unless he got a second opinion before admission, the insurer would only pay half. Astoundingly, Noah's plan even required a second opinion in the case of emergencies—if he was hit by a bus and taken to the hospital unconscious, he had to make sure the insurance company received a verifying medical opinion within twenty-four hours stating that he needed to be hospitalized, or they would simply deny half his costs! But because Noah didn't make this one simple phone call, he found himself saddled with a walloping medical bill at the end of his hospital stay—hardly the best medicine for his convalescence.

Noah's lesson holds true for many facets of insurance coverage. As costs rise, insurers are doing their best to scale back their coverage. They may act as drastically as they did for Noah and simply cut out half of what they pay. Or they may exclude a whole array of important benefits, such as home care, prescriptions, certain physicians' home visits, nursing, and diagnostic procedures. The result is that you fall into an insurance trap and you find out that you are less well covered than you expect.

Happily, the best prevention for this common problem is common sense. I suggest that you get up right now and go read your medical insurance policy. It is up to you to know what it contains. Don't assume, just because it was provided by a group, your company, or union, that you have adequate protection. Often, this simple exercise will alert you to hidden clauses—like the one Noah learned about the hard way—and hidden "catches" you have to know about in order to get the best possible coverage. Given the tremendous—and growing—role that insurance plays in your medical well-being, you owe it to yourself to be as well informed as possible about how to use it to your benefit.

## 6. Get Involved

My final counsel to you is a more general one. If you follow none of the above advice, I hope you'll take this one piece to heart. Starting right now, I hope you will resolve to become a more active participant in your own health care team. For the more involved you get, and the more committed you become, the greater your satisfaction, well-being, and overall health will be.

You may be saying to yourself, "But wait—I already take a real interest in my health. I've already made that commitment." I don't doubt that is true—after all, you are interested enough to be reading this book! But that doesn't mean there isn't more you could be doing. Perhaps you already exercise and watch what you eat, have stopped smoking, and feel comfortable speaking openly and directly with your doctor. Bravo! You still may want to ask yourself if there aren't areas where you could do even better, by becoming better informed or more involved.

Whether you are a novice or an old hand, I hope you will accept this book as a challenge to accept and renew your membership in your own health care team. You can become an active player in reshaping how our society views sickness and health, starting with your next visit to your doctor. I hope you accept my invitation to explore the cases and the symptomatology presented in the next chapters with an open mind, and so help educate yourself, your friends, and your family—and perhaps even your doctors.

If these pages do nothing other than to encourage you to make that commitment—and really follow through on it—they will have done their job.

# 5

# Phantom Diseases: Are *You* Falling Between the Cracks?

*"Since 1963, I have treated many patients with obvious diseases which can be seen by the naked eye or obviated by our sophisticated lab and X-ray examinations. I have also treated many patients with diseases and disorders which I could neither see with the naked eye, nor specifically obviate by these same examinations. I have labelled in good faith these many problems as: tension headache, fatigue syndrome, chronic ear infections, chronic sinusitis, irritable colon, depression, nerves, anxiety, situational reactions, hyperactive child syndrome, hypochondriasis, and nervous stomach. Some I even laid on the poor lowly virus. I thank God for viruses—even if I couldn't prove it so, the patient couldn't prove me wrong!"*

—Dr. Harold Hedges, M.D.
*Journal of the Arkansas Medical Society,*
Vol. 78, No. 8, January 1982, p. 336

*"There are no such things as incurables. There are only things for which Man has not found a cure."*

—Bernard Baruch

If you were to pick up and read several of the most prominent medical journals for even one month, I think you might be surprised at just how many of those pages are devoted to frank admissions of how very much we doctors still have to learn. Of course not all of them are as candid as the letter above, written to the editor of one such pro-

fessional review. But many of the submissions in those
pages touch on the same problem that Dr. Hedges alludes
to: our too-frequent ignorance and inability to give our
patients much more than a fancy name for what ails them,
while those same diseases and disorders sap their energy
and ruin their lives.

It is no accident that we have enshrined such ignorance
into our medical lexicon. If you need proof, you only have
to look at the whole basket of fancy, Latinate terms we
have coined to mask our shortcomings. We have *essential,*
as in *essential hypertension,* which means that the condition is just there and we don't know why. *Idiopathic* is
another such term, meaning "without known cause," as
is *cryptogenic.* Likewise, a whole dictionary of diagnoses,
a few of which Dr. Hedges refers to above, simply boil
down to names for things we don't understand.

Yet there is one term that you won't find in any medical
dictionary, or in any diagnostic textbook. It is what I call
the *phantom diseases.* These diseases are those that most
often manage to slip through the cracks of our medical
machine. Because of the vague, systemic, sporadic symptoms they can often produce—particularly in their early or
borderline cases—they form a whole class that is often
overlooked in the slam-bam high-tech-diagnostic way we
do medicine.

But that doesn't mean such diseases aren't very real—
and that they don't cause tremendous human suffering.
They most certainly do. A mother whose energy is sapped
and who cannot adequately care for her family, a father
whose job performance suffers because of annoying symptoms that are dragging him down, a student with severe
performance and learning problems caused by a hidden
condition—the list goes on and on. The truth is that when
it comes to suffering, there is no mystery at all about these
syndromes. They are very real, they can be very serious,
and the harm they do to millions of Americans is beyond
any reasonable dispute. Yet still the phantom diseases remain shadowy and elusive.

I christened them phantom after examining a patient who told me that she felt she was being haunted by a ghost. Donna had been persistently unhealthy for months, and visit after visit to a long string of doctors had revealed little seriously awry that could explain her severe symptoms. Yet she grew more listless, depressed, and withdrawn. Her mental processes and physical energy, she told me, "seemed all fogged up." In addition, she was gaining weight, and her once-youthful skin—for many years her pride—had become muddy and sallow. During her trips to my office, I diagnosed a borderline immune suppression and serious food intolerances. Once we began treatment, based on a strict dietary plan and nutrient supplements, she soon became like a woman reborn. Her skin cleared up, her energy rebounded to its prior exuberant levels, and the string of mental symptoms completely evaporated. "I feel great," she smiled, on her last visit. "Thank heaven that ghost has finally left me alone!"

What happened to Donna is typical of patients who suffer from phantom diseases—because these diseases often produce symptoms that easily fall between the diagnostic categories of our medical system.

## What Makes a Phantom?

The members of the phantom family share several traits in common. Perhaps the most significant hallmark is that, at least in the early stages, the problems often seem to come and go. Like the apparitions they are named for, phantom symptoms appear and disappear, as though written on shifting sands. One day you might be lethargic and barely able to get out of bed; the next, sunny and chipper, and a third somewhere in between. You may be fine for weeks, then suffer a string of bad days. These phantoms leave patients—and their loved ones—bothered, bewildered, to be sure, and also feeling bewitched. Needless to say, if your symptoms don't happen to occur just at the time when you are in your doctor's office, they can be damnably hard to pin down.

It is little wonder that this leads to one of the real tragedies of phantom diseases. Too often, when such an ongoing pattern gets established, patients—particularly women—may find themselves branded as "hypochondriac," manifesting "hysterical symptoms." Perhaps this is yet another form of medicalese that is too often invoked, simply a way of saying, "I can't find anything," and so taking the physician off the hook. I can't enumerate how many patients recount tales of being ignored, patronized, and pooh-poohed when they try to explain their vague problems. I can only think this happens because many practitioners aren't sufficiently acquainted with the many forms phantom diseases can take and the range of warning signs they can present in early or borderline cases.

A second hallmark of this nasty family of maladies is that they are notorious "sexists." That is to say, they take a disproportionate toll on women. In part this may be due to the greater biological complexity of the female animal, with its more intricate hormonal system. Several of these diseases, such as hypothyroidism, hypoglycemia, *Candida* infection, and premenstrual syndrome, appear to be intimately connected to our hormonal regulators, so it is not surprising that women are particularly at risk. To be sure, other members of the family prey more or less equally on both sexes. Such phantoms include labile hypertension, silent ischemic heart disease, and food sensitivities. But as a class, I would say that women represent an unfortunately high number of the victims of this family of disease. The sad irony is that often it is exactly this group of patients who are too easily dismissed by a medical establishment in which two-thirds of the practitioners are male.

The third trademark of phantom diseases is that their symptoms are usually systemic—that is, they involve the whole body, or several parts of it. Rarely do they produce a localized, specific ache or pain. If there is physical pain at all, it is likely to migrate throughout the body—in your joints, for example, in various parts of your digestive tract.

Much more commonly, symptoms involve overall body systems. You may feel that your energy, acuity, and mood is altered. You may know your digestion "isn't quite right" but not know what exactly is wrong. Your temperature regulation may suddenly seem thrown out of whack—feeling cold all the time, hot flashes, or chills. Because they work at such an insidious level, phantom diseases can affect everything we do, from eating and sleeping to exercise, work, and our sex lives. Through it all, the hallmark of phantom diseases is the broad, global dislocations they unleash.

People suffering from phantom diseases understand this all too well. They often present me with a complaint such as "Doctor Berger, I don't know what it is, but I know something's wrong. I am just not myself." When I hear that, I always assume that these patients are expressing a profound truth. After all, they are the ones living with their own body, every day and night. I operate from the assumption that few of them relish spending the time, money, and energy to jump from physician to physician. If they have made the effort to come into my office, I expect they are motivated by a true problem. And my first trail of inquiry is to make sure I don't overlook any phantom diseases.

This is closely tied to another distinctive characteristic of these phantoms. Not only do they present a potentially bewildering panoply of symptoms; often none of the symptoms they do create is terribly specific to the disease. Physicians who are used to treating conditions where "X symptom indicates Y disorder" often find themselves at sea when the phantoms rear their heads. Because these diseases usually do their work in telltale patterns, their diagnosis depends on recognizing conjunctions of mutually occurring symptoms. They require diagnosis by viewing the forest, not the trees. Because phantoms resist neat, tidy, one-to-one diagnoses, they often frustrate physician and patient alike.

The way phantom diseases get to be phantoms is that they are too often ignored by our medical practitioners. Particularly when they occur in a borderline situation, they usually demand significant diagnostic sophistication in order to be unearthed. The doctor may have to assess environment, life-style, heredity, and chemical and psychological stressors to bring these phantoms to light. Not surprisingly, unless a physician is acutely aware of just what he or she is looking for, it is possible to miss the subtle clues that a phantom is at work. As a result, you may not undergo the full-scale, in-depth profiling you require . . . and the shadowy phantom slides by, undetected.

It is my credo that the single best way to make sure you are not a victim of these problems is by giving you the information your doctor may not have, and the confidence you need, to rule them out. Thus, this section is geared to providing helpful information you can put to use *now*.

## Meet the Phantoms

Of course, almost any medical condition—from mumps to allergies—can at times behave like a phantom. That is, it can be elusive, hard to pin down, or create broad, subtle problems. But that does not mean it should properly be classed as a phantom.

What distinguishes the true phantom diseases is not just that they *can* be difficult to track down or that they are sometimes easy to overlook. What distinguishes them is that that is their very nature. They make a habit of being elusive. These diseases simply won't be found unless your doctor is conscientiously and systematically looking for them, looking hard, and in the right places with the right tools. It is no great surprise that these are the syndromes most likely to ''slip through the cracks.''

Who are they? Meet the phantoms:

- The silent curse of hypothyroidism, which, authorities estimate, affects some ten million Americans
- Hidden ischemic cardiac disease, which, according to Harvard University scientists, is a deadly precursor to fatal heart attacks, yet is not recognized except under specific conditions
- Hidden, chronic infections of the yeast organism *(Candida albicans)*, usually overlooked by medical practitioners
- The often-discussed, but too-little-recognized, symptoms of hypoglycemia (low blood sugar), which can affect one's energy, psychological functioning, mental alertness, and general organ health
- The slippery, elusive blood pressure disorder labile hypertension, which today puts 36 million Americans at risk for stroke, cardiovascular disease, and grave kidney problems
- Hidden food sensitivities, affecting some tens of millions of Americans, which can disturb every facet of your physical and psychological health, disrupt your immune balance, and put you at risk for immune diseases
- Premenstrual syndromes, conservatively estimated to create significant medical and emotional problems for forty million women in this country every month

Other experts might well include different phantoms, but it is my firm belief that, by themselves, the diseases just listed account for more than 90 percent of what can properly be termed phantom diseases. To be sure, they are a motley, and a dangerous, crew of illnesses. But happily, they can be vanquished with a combination of up-to-date knowledge, keen observation, and persistent dedication—both yours and your doctor's.

## Get Your Fair Share

*"The world has become crowded with knowledge, and there is more to come. The fair distribution of knowledge will be a more important problem in the century ahead than at any time in the past."*
— Dr. Lewis Thomas, chairman,
Memorial Sloan-Kettering Cancer Institute

In no domain are those words more prescient than in the area of medical research and discovery, and I think they make a fitting end for this chapter. With all the phantom diseases, the fact is that unless your doctor is uncommonly well versed in the many forms these masqueraders can take, there is a strong likelihood that you will personally have an important role to play in the maintenance of your own health. You may have to bring new findings on the subject to his or her attention or you may want to do extra reading to rule out possibilities; you may even want to suggest certain tests or procedures and get your doctor's thoughts about them. That is the "fair distribution" Dr. Thomas wrote about—the fact that it is not just your physician, but you, who must know what's what if you are to chase these phantoms out of your life once and for all.

I should add here one point that I hope is already obvious. The point of the following chapters is in no way meant to replace, second-guess, compete with, or undermine your own relationship with your family or personal doctor. That would be both unhelpful and unwise. Instead, I hope you view these chapters as a supplement to the most successful care. The idea is to bring you as a partner into the medical decision-making—and even fact-finding—process.

For that reason, in many of the following chapters I have included a section entitled "For Deeper Study," listing other resources where you can go if you want to learn more about a particular problem or issue. You may, for example, suspect that the phantom of hypoglycemia is particularly relevant to you or someone close to you. At the end of that chapter, you'll find tips for resources where you can look to deepen your understanding.

Sometimes you will find that I have recommended books or magazine articles, other times information agencies or medical societies that specialize in one area or another. All of them, of course, are optional. There's no pressure, and no, there won't be a quiz! But together, I hope these resources let you take your knowledge one step further.

It is my deepest wish that by pointing the way to further discovery, these chapters will give you the tools to vanquish the phantoms that may now be plaguing you and your family. So, now that you have made the acquaintance of these phantoms as a group, let's take them on, one by one.

# 6

# Hypothyroidism:
# When Your Energy Thermostat
# Breaks Down

I can think of no more clear-cut example of the toll phantom diseases take on our nation's well-being than the millions of people who suffer under the shadow of hidden hypothyroidism. Alarmingly widespread and grossly underrecognized, this stealthily creeping disease can have profound implications for your energy, vitality, and overall mental and physical health.

Yet behind its technical-sounding name is a relatively straightforward disorder. Simply put, what happens is that your thyroid gland, which is responsible for your body's metabolism, becomes sluggish. As it does so, it curtails production of its essential thyroid hormones. That simple change sends ripples throughout virtually every system and organ in your body. But to understand all it can mean, it's necessary to understand something about how your thyroid works when you are well and all that it does to keep you strong and vital.

Your thyroid is a small, walnut-size gland weighing about an ounce and situated in your neck, just below your Adam's apple.

## Find Your Thyroid

Seen from the front, your thyroid looks like a small, butterfly-shaped gland, with each "wing" nestling around either side of your windpipe. You can locate it by feeling with your fingers about an inch below your Adam's apple. If you feel directly below the point of the Adam's apple you'll feel a harder, ridged section—your windpipe, or trachea. Following that down about an inch, you'll feel it give way to a softer, more pliable section. That is where the thin band of your thyroid crosses the windpipe and where its two lobes straddle the trachea on either side. Most likely, you won't feel anything much there, but don't worry, that's as it should be. If you felt a hard, clearly delineated growth or a tender or resistant organ, that could be a sign that you may have something wrong.

Your body's glands go, it is a relatively simple one, for its primary duty is to produce two hormones: triiodothyronine and thyroxine (physicians usually call them $T_3$ and $T_4$, respectively, for brevity's sake). These two crucial hormones travel to organs throughout the body—including your heart, liver, brain, and kidneys—where they regulate how fast your bodily processes go. The higher your levels of circulating thyroid hormone, the more "revved up" all your body's systems become—that is, your organs and cells burn the oxygen and sugar they use for fuel more rapidly. In effect, the level of thyroid hormone you have sets the idling speed for your entire body.

Usually, that level stays in careful balance, because your thyroid gland responds to chemical instructions from your pituitary gland. But sometimes, your carefully tuned levels of $T_3$ and $T_4$ fall out of balance. If you have too much of the hormones in your blood (a condition called *hyper—*

"over"—*thyroidism*), your organs and muscles burn up calories (energy) faster, your heart speeds up, you become nervous, jumpy, and hungry, and your digestive processes and bowel movements speed up. Like a race car burning a too-rich fuel mixture, you run faster than nature "tuned" you to do, and the symptoms that develop are those of a body running too fast.

But much more common is the reverse problem: hypothyroidism, (*hypo* meaning "under"—that is underproduction of thyroid hormone, or *HT* for short). In this case, the symptoms are just the opposite. In fact, as one patient, a mechanic, very accurately put it, it's like "someone watered my gas tank." You feel heavy, slow-starting, and severely lacking in energy. All your faculties—mind, memory, and emotions—seem dulled. You get a sleepy, sluggish feeling. As the condition becomes more pronounced, symptoms may show up in virtually every area of your body: skin, hair, mood, even your body's ability to conceive a child. In short, it feels as if your biological processes are slowly petering out.

You may also hear the disease referred to by its more clinical name, myxedema, which is usually reserved for serious, advanced hypothyroidism. But whatever the label, HT is an archetypal phantom disease, one that takes an enormous cost in terms of human suffering and illness yet is often very hard to pin down.

## What's *Your* Risk?

It is certainly true that this disease takes a tremendous toll on millions of people in our country. But its damage comes not so much because it takes a huge toll on any one person. Rather, it is the number of people it affects, not its severity for any one individual, that makes it such a serious health problem. In fact, one reason HT conditions are so widespread—and so widely overlooked—is because it is not a killer, rarely dramatic in its effects, and creates no sudden disruptions in people's lives. Instead, it does its damage stealthily, taking a gradual, insidious toll on the energy, stability, and vitality of many millions of us.

Just how widespread is the problem? One recent book reports that as many as *one in four* adult Americans suffer from some degree of hypothyroidism. Another physician, a man who spent his professional life studying the thyroid gland and its effects, places the figure much higher—up to 40 percent of adult Americans with some degree of thyroid impairment. If these numbers are even remotely accurate, that makes 96 million Americans whose lives are hampered in some way with unnecessary fatigue and hypothyroid symptoms. There can be no doubt: we are suffering from a national pandemic of silent, phantom thyroid disease.

Yet even if you take the most conservative figures, there is clear cause for concern. Dr. Lawrence Wood, instructor at Harvard Medical School and president of the Thyroid Foundation of America, estimates that some *eight to ten million* Americans suffer from thyroid disorders. To put that into perspective, even if this rock-bottom estimate is true, it means that more people suffer from this phantom illness than from coronary heart disease and cancer *combined.* I find it interesting that, alongside the deluge of publicity surrounding those "media" diseases, the silence around our pandemic of hypothyroidism is truly deafening. Of course, it is not as dramatic, but there is little argument that the subtle, chronic problems of HT take a tremendous toll on the quality of life of millions of Americans every day. Nevertheless, it remains largely unrecognized, consigned to the shadows of a phantom illness.

## The Great Imposter

Probably the main reason that HT is so often overlooked is that it so readily mimics the symptoms of many other diseases. In this it resembles a biological chameleon, making itself appear first like one problem, then like another. The whole time the hapless thyroid sufferer may shuttle from one specialist to the next in a vain effort to track down what is wrong. Of course, this only adds to the frustration and emotional devastation that low thyroid can mean for its sufferers.

By definition, we will never know just how many cases of HT go undetected each year. But it has been estimated by Harvard University's Dr. Lawrence Wood that as many as one-fifth of the victims of low thyroid are sick enough to be on medication, yet remain either undiagnosed or misdiagnosed.

Such misdiagnoses can take many forms. Commonly, the fatigue and lethargy of HT mimics the clinical signs of depression, and it is not uncommon for people to find themselves saddled with a diagnosis of mental illness. They may get put on strong drugs, including mood elevators and antidepressants, when, in fact, it is not their brain chemistry but their thyroid that is at fault. This is a particular problem for women, not only because women are four times more likely than men to suffer from thyroid disorders in the first place, but because many physicians are quick to label women as suffering from "hysterical" symptoms when they can find nothing obviously wrong.

Similarly, according to a study from New Jersey's Biopsychiatry Center, reported in the *New England Journal of Medicine*, thyroid problems in women are often misdiagnosed as premenstrual syndrome. That study suggested that as many as *two-thirds* of PMS diagnoses may in fact reflect subclinical thyroid disorders.

Sometimes, these misdiagnoses lead to real medical blunders. I have even read unconfirmed reports of cases where women have undergone radical hysterectomies because of abnormally heavy menstrual bleeding. But when surgery failed to correct the condition, it has been found that the bleeding was due to hypothyroidism all along and that once that underlying condition was corrected, the heavy bleeding subsided.

Needless drugs, damaging diagnoses, unnecessary surgery—as you can see, the toll of this particular phantom disease reaches far beyond its own symptoms. The lesson here is that the best defense is a good offense. For you, that means knowing whether you are a candidate for HT, what its symptoms are, and what you can do about them.

## Thyroid-Risk Profile

Happily, one of the best weapons we have against the phantom of hidden hypothyroidism is that the risk groups are fairly clear-cut. That means, of course, that certain kinds of people are much more likely to suffer from this problem than are others. The first step is to check yourself out. Do you fit into the profile below?

• Are you female? (Women are four times more likely than men to have low thyroid.)
• Are you past menopause? (HT tends to occur in women after age fifty or so.)
• Are you taking lithium? (The drug can cause both hypo- and hyper-thyroid problems.)
• Have you ever had radiation treatments near your neck region? (This can cause delayed damage to the thyroid gland.)
• Did you have a grandparent with thyroid problems? (Thyroid disorders may run in families, skipping a generation.)
• If you are a woman, did you have noticeable gray hair before the age of thirty? (Premature graying in females appears to have a genetic link to low-thyroid problems.)

If you don't find yourself here, it doesn't necessarily mean you are completely out of danger. With this disease, as with so many things in medicine, statistics can be deceptive. Gregory Z. was a perfect case of that. According to the books, Greg was in no high-risk group for HT. Just thirty-four years old, this young man had, until recently, been in top health. But when he came to me, one look told me that something was clearly very wrong.

"A couple of years ago, I started my own computer business," he explained. "Everything was great—growing, expanding, I had a great time." His words, I noticed, were labored, heavy. "But then something happened. I started feeling weak, you know—just lazier than I was used to feeling. Now it's been six months or so, and I just haven't felt . . . like myself." I clearly heard the weariness in his voice. "I used to go nonstop all day and still feel terrific by evening. Now I go home exhausted—it's just not right to feel this tired."

At first, he explained, he thought it might be some emotional problems that he was wrestling with, but soon realized they could not account for his increasing lethargy. Then the truth hit: Whatever was going on was a cause, not a result, of his blue feelings. The other concern, he told me in a small voice, was that his sexual performance—and interest—had trailed off to almost zero. "It's not even something I look forward to anymore. I'd rather sleep."

A trip to his regular doctor turned up nothing. After a battery of tests, Gregory was pronounced "perfectly healthy," and advised to take a vacation. He did, but came back almost as tired as when he left. Desperate, he tried a psychiatrist, but after six months, realized there was little improvement. "I'm starting to feel as if I have a terrible terminal disease that nobody's telling me about," he admitted as he slouched in the chair opposite me.

His constellation of symptoms suggested HT, so I ran the necessary tests, including a specialized body-temperature test that can often be more sensitive to thyroid problems than standard laboratory blood tests. The result pointed clearly to a borderline thyroid deficiency, so I put Gregory on a regime of thyroid medication.

Two months later, I hardly recognized the perky Greg, who bounded into my waiting room. There was a new glow about him. "This is just like my old self," he smiled. His depression and lethargy had lifted completely, and his symptoms—constantly feeling cold, excessive fatigue—had evaporated. "There's a great side benefit, too," he winked. "Sex has never been better." The moral of Gregory's tale is a simple one: the phantom of HT can haunt anyone, even if you're not in the high-risk group.

## Do You Show These Signs?

More important by far than the statistics of an illness are its symptoms. The truth is that, from your perspective as a health-interested person, the question is not who usually gets the illness according to the statistics but *whether it is indeed happening to you.* You are not a biostatistician, you are an individual.

Happily, I have two relatively simple and foolproof ways you can answer this question for yourself. Of course, you are welcome to use these techniques to help others besides yourself. It is my fondest wish that you will put them to work to assess the health of your spouse or lover, of your children, your parents, and even your friends. I like to think, in fact, that if everybody who reads this book were to be vigilant about how this disease touches simply those in his or her own personal circle, we could help drive this phantom disease out of the closet once and for all!

The first of the two techniques is simple. On the following page is a screening checklist for the signs and symptoms that might indicate hypothyroid (myxedema) conditions.

## Two Steps to Health:
## The Thyroid Screening Self-Check

|  | True | False |
|---|---|---|
| 1. I have had unaccustomed problems with constipation. | ____ | ____ |
| 2. I seem to get cold more often than I used to. | ____ | ____ |
| 3. My hands and feet, especially, get cold easily. | ____ | ____ |
| 4. I notice I often feel tired and fatigued. | ____ | ____ |
| 5. There is a rounded swelling at the base of my neck. | ____ | ____ |
| 6. My memory seems to be weaker than it used to be. | ____ | ____ |
| 7. My voice has taken on a husky, hoarse quality or has deepened recently. | ____ | ____ |
| 8. My skin feels rougher and coarser than usual. | ____ | ____ |
| 9. My face and eyes look or feel puffy. | ____ | ____ |
| 10. I generally feel slower, more sluggish than normal. | ____ | ____ |
| 11. I am sleeping noticeably more than usual. | ____ | ____ |
| 12. I have noticed that I am less alert, retentive, or concentrate less well than usual. | ____ | ____ |
| 13. I gain weight markedly more than I did a year ago. | ____ | ____ |
| 14. I have a prolonged menstrual period, with quite significant bleeding. | ____ | ____ |
| 15. My hair has been falling out more easily. | ____ | ____ |
| 16. My skin seems uncommonly dry and flaky. | ____ | ____ |
| 17. I've felt blue and depressed recently. | ____ | ____ |
| 18. I have noticed various muscle cramps lately. | ____ | ____ |
| 19. I have been having recurrent headaches. | ____ | ____ |
| 20. I find myself drinking more coffee, teas, or caffeine-containing colas to boost my energy. | ____ | ____ |
| 21. I suspect I may have a fertility problem. | ____ | ____ |

Obviously, many of these are common symptoms and are hard to pin down and quantify accurately. What really counts is not the presence of any one, but a conjunction of several of them. If you answered yes to any five of the above, it could well mean that you have "passed" through the initial screen—that is, that you have a reasonable chance of suffering from HT. Your own situation may range from almost nonexistent to borderline or even quite significant, so the important next step is to pinpoint more accurately which is the case.

## Second Step: Take the Barnes Test

Pinning down this diagnosis is easily done with step two of this process. It is called the Barnes Basal Metabolism Test, and it was developed by Dr. Broda Barnes, a researcher and physician who spent much of his professional life researching and writing extensively on low thyroid. In fact, if there is any one man responsible for our current understanding of the profound and extensive implications of hypothyroidism, it is Dr. Barnes.

Many years ago, realizing the need for a simple, safe, noninvasive screen for thyroid problems, Dr. Barnes developed an easy, do-at-home test. It is based on the fact that when the thyroid begins to slow your body down, one of the first signs is a drop in your overall temperature. It makes sense—after all, if you have a low level of thyroid hormones $T_3$ and $T_4$, your body's energy furnaces are essentially being banked. That loss in energy means that you are running a little "cooler." The Barnes Test determines this by charting your overall body temperature.

Many doctors protest that this Barnes Test is not sufficiently precise, because it relies upon such a broad, systemic sign as temperature, which can be affected by so many diverse factors. My answer to this is that of course it isn't foolproof—not by itself. But a positive result combined with some of the frank symptoms listed above is certainly suggestive enough that it makes it worthwhile consulting your own doctor.

That makes the Barnes Test the best thing I know to recommend to patients who are concerned that they may have HT. After all, the true goal of patient-centered, preventive medicine is not that all of us become world-class diagnostic technicians. It is that we become alert to the early signs and symptoms and know when we ought to seek professional help. The most august medical authorities agree about this when the problems concern your heart or pancreas, as in diabetes or cancer—so why, I ask, does it not apply equally when the problem concerns your thyroid gland?

So, if the step-one screen raises some questions for you, I suggest you invest forty-three minutes into this easy step-two test. If you come out positive, I'll discuss, below, what your next reasonable step should be.

## The Barnes Test

1. Place a standard oral fever thermometer within easy reach at your bedside before you go to sleep tonight.
2. Tomorrow, when you awaken, immediately put the thermometer in either armpit and keep it there for five minutes. Record your temperature, then get up and go about your day.
3. Repeat this for fourteen days, every day, recording your temperature each day. This is done for two weeks to rule out any chance fluctuation due to illness.
   (Special note for women: To obtain the most accurate results, the test must be performed during the period when you are not menstruating.)
4. If, at the end of the two-week sampling period, you show a consistent pattern of low temperature—that is, below 98 degrees—*and* you suffer from any of the signs listed in step one, I suggest you may want to bring up the subject of HT with your own doctor. One special note: A positive result on the Barnes Test is particularly

suggestive if you know that your body doesn't customarily run a subnormal (low) body temperature.

If you are concerned after taking these tests, the next step is fairly clear-cut: Consult your doctor. It is up to her or him to do the standard, simple blood measurements that are most often used to diagnose hypothyroid. But you notice I said "fairly" clear-cut. That's because there is a distinct possibility that some doctors may not be aware of the newest technologies to unearth subtle or borderline HT.

## Give Your Doctor a Hand

Two decades ago, when many of the doctors in practice were trained, the standard thyroid tests were crude and insensitive. The only tests were for the thyroid hormones themselves—$T_3$ and $T_4$. In those days, many patients with real, chronic low-thyroid problems were sent home with a diagnosis of malingering because the medical assays weren't sensitive enough to pick up their very real biochemical problem. The problem was put in a nutshell by one practicing physician in the pages of the *Journal of the American Medical Association:* "The primary reason for overlooking hypothyroidism is the placing of too much reliance on a single metabolic test. Such a test rarely registers lower than it should, in contrast to frequent false-high readings."

Happily, today, your doctor has much more powerful tools available. Your physician now knows—or certainly should—that it is not just enough to look at whether your $T_3$ and $T_4$ hormones are low. A more revealing test measures your blood levels of thyroid-stimulating hormone, or TSH. This chemical messenger is released from your pituitary gland and is what carries the instruction to your thyroid to produce its hormones in the first place.

TSH comes from the pituitary gland, where it is released when that gland senses there is not enough of the thyroid hormone in the blood. The TSH works to tell your thyroid to "turn up the production." So if your pituitary senses a chronic low level of thyroid hormones, it tries to awaken the thyroid by sending its message more loudly—that is, by sending out more TSH. A high level of TSH in your blood suggests that the correct biological message is being sent, but that your thyroid is not listening to it. That may be an early warning sign that there are thyroid problems ahead. Not surprisingly, many experts feel that this assay is the single best way to pinpoint subtle or incipient cases of HT.

If neither of the above tests shows anything, it may mean that you're perfectly okay, or it may mean that you have a very borderline case of "tired thyroid." To rule that out, I suggest you ask your doctor about the advisability of taking one other kind of test, the TRH test.

Believe me, if you take all of these screens and nothing untoward shows up, you can be fairly certain your thyroid is definitely doing its best to keep you healthy. If you continue to experience the symptoms listed in step one, I suggest you look elsewhere for the cause of your complaints.

It may sound like a lot of tests, but the thyroid battery is quite accurate, relatively inexpensive, and no more painful than the minor needle prick it takes to draw blood. When you balance that against the dreary prospect of living life under a low-thyroid cloud, believe me, it is a prudent and worthwhile investment. But again, only you can determine that, by using the two-step process as I outlined above.

## Ready for the Silver Lining?

You have already heard the bad news about HT, seen how it hides, and learned of the tremendous systemic symptoms it can wreak throughout your body. I know it may sound a little bleak, but take heart, there is some good news here as well. The good news is something virtually every clinician will agree on: Once diagnosed, hypothyroidism is relatively simple and straightforward to fix. Our medical machine may not always do very well at finding this phantom in the first place, but once we do, we understand very well how to go about exorcising it.

If you are found to have clinically demonstrable low thyroid, your doctor will put you on a simple thyroid booster, made of a synthetic form of thyroid hormone. The medicine is available in easy-to-take pills, which you will have to take every day. You should expect that it will take a little time and effort to adjust the dosage at first. But once that has been done, most people stay on these pills with a minimum of side effects and bother and can do so indefinitely without complications. With this phantom, the hard part is bringing it to light. Once you and your doctor have done that, you can expect treatment to be easy, safe, and relatively risk-free.

## Be on Guard

Even if you are not one who exhibits the symptoms of low thyroid, it may pay to be a little vigilant, because there are things you can do to help lower your risk for HT. In spite of much research, it remains true that the exact mechanisms that create low-thyroid problems remain as cloudy and elusive as the symptoms of the disease itself.

We know that one of the most common causes involves the mineral iodine. By this I don't mean the red liquid you dab on a cut finger, but the vital micronutrient found in many different kinds of foods. Your thyroid depends heavily on the iodine you ingest, for without the mineral it cannot synthesize its thyroid hormones. Not surprisingly, in many parts of the world where iodine is scarce, people suffer from thyroid imbalances. In its most dramatic form, it can cause the massive swellings on the neck known as goiter, which you may have seen in photographs taken in developing countries.

In this country it is uncommon for people to show signs

of too little iodine. It is recommended that we get about 300 micrograms of iodine each day, but most Americans consume about twice that in our daily diets. It comes to you, hidden, from many sources: shellfish and seafood, certain mushrooms, the water you drink, and the iodized salt you eat. Between them all, it is likely that you get your daily share—and then some.

Where problems can arise is if you suddenly increase how much iodine you get. Suppose you acquire a taste for kelp or seaweed products, which are extremely rich sources of iodine. It may sound unlikely, but many health food fanciers, as well as sushi devotees, can actually get a significant dose of iodine this way. It comes not just from seaweed products themselves but from the fresh fish and shellfish eaten with them. The result of such an increase can be to throw off your body's careful iodine balance and kick off a cycle of hypothyroidism. In fact, abruptly changing your iodine intake has the potential both to lower and to raise your thyroid's activity. Ironically, this can happen when people decide to start eating better and add significant amounts of new, seemingly "healthy" foods to their diets—foods such as kelp and seaweed preparations.

Obviously, there is nothing wrong per se with eating these foods, but it must be done in moderation, building them up in your diet slowly. Equally clear is that eating ocean products does not in itself account for the millions of cases of phantom hypothyroid disease. Scientists believe there are many possible causes for low thyroid. I divide these causes into two groups.

The first are the "inevitables"—that is, there is little you can do about them. They may involve your genetic makeup. It has been noted that women with premature graying also seem to have a strong chance of thyroid imbalance. If correct, that is strong evidence for a gene-based predisposition to thyroid weakness. The more we learn about the thyroid-gene link, the better, more accurate job we will do of diagnosing which people should be especially carefully examined for thyroid disease.

Also in this category are the thyroid problems due to autoimmune processes. In that case, your body's internal regulatory mechanisms actually start to attack the thyroid gland, eventually crippling its own hormone production. Like the genetic hypothesis, there is little you can currently do to safeguard yourself against this immune imbalance.

But the second group of possible causes for thyroid problems holds greater cause for optimism, because you *can* do something about them. Physicians are looking into factors such as stress as a possible factor in thyroid imbalance. Although the medical jury is still out, this may add yet another reason why all of us should engage in stress-reduction activities on a regular basis. It is also thought that factors such as radiation, certain medicines, and even foods may play a role in thyroid functioning.

## Eating for a Healthy Thyroid

Probably the most prudent thing you can do to make sure your thyroid stays in balance is to make sure it has all the nutrients it needs. We have already talked about the importance of keeping stable and reasonable amounts of iodine in your food. For my patients, I recommend they just make sure to keep an adequate supply of iodine-rich foods in their diets—foods such as seafood, cereals, and some fruits and vegetables. As we saw earlier, people in this country rarely suffer from iodine deficiencies.

But new research suggests that there are other factors to consider, as well, in order to keep your thyroid ticking along happily. We know that your thyroid needs adequate levels of vitamins including A, C, E, and $B_2$ (thiamine). Minerals play an equally important role, especially minerals such as zinc and selenium. Preliminary research from Japan suggests that people with low thyroid manifest an imbalance of notably depressed levels of zinc in their blood, especially in their red blood cells. Another paper, from the *American Journal of Clinical Nutrition*, suggests that low zinc impairs your thyroid's ability to produce its crucial hormones. The relationship between vital micronutrients and thyroid—whether low zinc helps cause thyroid disease or is the result of a disordered thyroid—is complex and not yet fully understood. But it does seem clear that if your thyroid lacks any of this crucial nutrient, it runs a greater likelihood of becoming sluggish and failing to secrete the necessary thyroid hormones to keep you vital, healthy, and alert. So, for all of us it makes sense to build adequate zinc into what we eat. That means eating foods such as whole grains, nuts, seafood, wheat germ, and bran.

While we're on the subject of mineral supplements, I have one, very important, special word just for women. Women thyroid sufferers who are pregnant should *avoid excess iodine at all costs*. We now know that too much iodine can cause a number of thyroid-related problems in the developing fetus, from hypothyroidism to goiter. In general, iodine should *not* be a part of a prenatal supplementation regimen, and it is probably well advised to avoid a diet chocked full of iodine-saturated foods.

Eventually, it seems clear that as we learn more, we will discover that robust and stable thyroid health depends on an intricate balance of factors and that changing any one of these can result in the creeping symptoms of chronic hypothyroidism. For the moment, eating well, reducing stress, and keeping acutely attuned to your body's subtle thyroid signals are probably the best ways to give yourself built-in protection against hypothyroid disorders.

## For Deeper Study

If you want to know more about thyroid disorders, or need to know where to get help, here are some extra resources my patients have found very helpful:

Lawrence Wood, M.D. *Your Thyroid: A Home Reference.* New York: Ballantine Books, 1986.

Stephen E. Langer, M.D. *Solved: The Riddle of Illness*. New York: Keats Publishing, 1984.

"A Closer Look at Your Thyroid." Travenol Laboratories, Flint Division, Deerfield, Illinois 60015 (1983).

American Thyroid Association, Mayo Clinic, 200 First Street, S.W., Rochester, Minnesota 55905. Tel. (507) 284-4738.

The Thyroid Foundation of America, c/o Lawrence Wood, M.D., 535 Ambulatory Care Center, Massachusetts General Hospital, Boston, Massachusetts 02114.

The Thyroid Foundation of Canada, P.O. Box 1643, Kingston, Ontario K7L5C8. Tel. (613) 546-1576.

# 7

# The Phantom Yeast: The Candida Connection

For most of us, the word *yeast* conjures up all sorts of homey, nutritious images. We associate it with the smell of a loaf of bread rising in the oven, the taste of delicious fresh cookie dough, or the pleasure of a cool glass of beer on a hot summer's day.

But behind such benign associations lurks a darker side to this "friendly" yeast. Every day, that side causes untold pain, suffering, and frustration for many millions of Americans. In most cases it does so stealthily, silently, without us even being aware of it. It is what I call the Yeast Beast, and it is one of most common and most serious of phantom diseases.

Like most people, you probably think of yeast as something that comes in the supermarket, in powder or compressed cakes—the stuff bakers use to make bread, rolls, and cakes rise. As far as it goes, that's true.

But the biological fact is that yeast is a beast. The tasty stuff you eat in rolls, breads, and beer is, scientifically, alive. In biological terms, the yeast is termed a unicellular microorganism—a tiny, one-celled living animal—that lives, breathes, and reproduces. In fact, when your grandmother put yeast into a bowl of warm water and sugar to start a loaf of bread, she was giving it an ideal culture in which to reproduce—and as it began to proliferate, the by-products of its reproductive process are what made her breads and baked goods rise.

106

## Not a Nice Family . . .

There are a whole family of yeasts, but the ones that cause the most trouble in the body consist of a relatively distinct quartet: *Candida albicans, Candida glabrata, Candida tropicalis, and Candida parapsilosis.* But most of these don't create a lot of infection problems in humans. Far and away the greatest number of yeast infections can be laid at the feet (if it had any) of one particularly nasty member of the yeast family: *Candida albicans.*

When it comes to finding these tiny animals, you don't have to look far. *Candida* organisms are omnipresent in the environment—in the air you breathe, the wool sweater you wear, in damp corners, on carpets, in much of what we drink and eat. Not surprisingly, these aggressive microscopic spores aren't just outside you. They also live inside you, in the innermost reaches of your digestive tract and other organs, on a permanent basis.

Starting when you were a small baby, yeasts were some of the first residents to take up lodging inside you. You got them from the air, from fruit juices and foods, even from the nipples of your bottles. In fact, it was those same fungal yeast infections that caused the diaper rash you probably had (even if you don't quite remember it today!).

From the yeast's-eye-view, you represent a vast, safe continent to colonize, providing warm, specialized nooks and crevices where they can live and breed in happy splendor. As you read these words, yeast colonies are thriving, multiplying, and dying, in your digestive tract, your rectum, your vagina (if you're a woman), on your skin, and perhaps even in your mouth.

Most of the time, yeast remains a benign biological tenant. So long as it has a comfy place to live and reproduce, it stays controlled and happy. Normally, in the exquisite homeostasis maintained within a healthy human body, your yeast is kept in line by legions of other organisms, which compete for nutrients and prey on the yeast, thereby keeping it confined in well-ordered, tightly controlled, biological niches.

But sometimes—alarmingly often, as we will see—something goes awry. Then, like some gruesome Stephen King novel, those homey, pleasant guests turn into something quite vicious. When the careful balance keeping yeast organisms in check is disrupted, yeast colonies can grow out of control and may flare into a severe local infection.

You may have had this happen already if you are one of the millions of women who have had vaginal yeast infections. But such infections can also occur in the rectum, on the skin, or even in your mouth, where a *Candida* infection coats the tongue with a white, sticky layer and is termed *thrush*.

But sometimes, in what is termed *Candida overgrowth*, the yeast breaks out of local infections and goes on a rampage, an out-of-control riot. Under certain biological conditions in your body, *Candida* changes from a simple, relatively benign yeast form into what is called a *mycelial fungal* form.

In that state, it begins to spread out from its usual niche in your gastrointestinal tract, sending out tentaclelike growths into the walls of your intestines, where it can come into direct contact with your bloodstream. Once in contact with the blood, yeasts can liberate chemical waste products from their reproduction.

Now, those yeast by-products may help a cake rise, but they don't help your bloodstream. In fact, it is believed that these products act like toxins, creating serious symptoms in virtually every system of your body. Hence the wide and bewildering range of symptoms attributed to yeast infections.

## What's in a Name?

The dangerous yeast overgrowth that can cause such symptoms goes by many names. Your physician may term it alternatively *candidiasis* or *moniliasis,* after the medical name for the yeast organism. Popular books often term it simply *yeast overgrowth*. Other times, you may see it referred to as polysystemic chronic candidiasis, or PCC, to distinguish it from more localized yeast infections. I have also heard it called yeast poisoning, because of the overwhelming toxic load that an overabundance of *Candida* organisms puts on your body. I prefer the term PCC, because it reminds us that it is a chronic and poly-system ("many" system) disease. But whatever you choose to call it, the fact is that when yeast gets beastly, the results can be terrible indeed.

Nobody knows that better than one of my patients, Dr. B. At fifty-seven years old, Dr. B. had a distinguished career as a psychotherapist spanning three decades. But recently, something had started going wrong. It began with a persistent skin rash, causing irritating itching and burning. But soon the rash-covered areas began to swell, and Dr. B. started running fevers with no explainable cause.

Worse, whatever he had started affecting his mental state. He found himself feeling impatient and irritable with his clients, his body's agony dulling the keen interpersonal edge he needed to maintain his practice. Meanwhile, his rash seemed to spread every day, and now it had covered almost all of his body. It became so overwhelming, and the itching so painful and maddening, that Dr. B. was forced to reduce, and then eliminate, his practice.

A practicing professional, Dr. B. knew he needed qualified expert advice, so he brought himself to New York City to see the best doctor he could find. That dermatologist put him in the hospital for ten days of exhaustive, exhausting, and expensive tests. But when all was done, the result was nothing more than a label: atopic dermatitis—one of those catchall diagnoses for a skin condition that physicians do not know how to cure.

"Finally, they threw up their hands," recalls Dr. B., with a trace of bitterness. "They simply didn't know what to do." They told him they could give him prednisone, a cortisonelike drug that would reduce his immediate symptoms of swelling and itching. But he could not stay on such a toxic drug indefinitely without risking much more serious problems. "In other words," he explained, "the doctors told me, I couldn't survive without prednisone, and I couldn't survive with it." As I sat facing this doctor on his first visit, it was clear that he was a man in agony and despair.

His profile—several hypersensitivities, including corn and polyesters, asthma, and elevated blood pressure and cholesterol—suggested some systemic phantom illness. The tests I gave him pointed to *Candida* infection as the culprit, so I prescribed a strict dietary plan. The first step was to remove the sources of yeast spore in the food he ate every day and so avoid exacerbating an already-bad situation. Next, we would rebuild his immune system, following the program I outlined in my book, *Dr. Berger's Immune Power Diet.*

Because of his yeast problem, I prescribed a diet free of bread and baked products containing yeast and free of alcohol, mushrooms, and fermented foods. In addition, because of the antibiotics often used in processing it, I warned him away from the red meats that were a favorite part of his diet.

The results were overwhelming. When he returned six weeks later, his worst symptoms had clearly abated. For the first time in months, he was able to sleep and work comfortably, since the maddening itching and swelling was disappearing. The progress was reflected in his laboratory tests, which showed that his blood pressure had dropped to a textbook-perfect 120/80. Dr. B. looked over my shoulder at one of his tests, showing that the ratio of his immune-helper cells to immune-suppressor cells—an indicator of overall immune health—had already risen by more than two points. Other measures of allergic activity had gone from being off the scale to being well within normal range.

But best of all was how he felt. "I'm back to my old self," he smiled. A month later, he called me back with a sheepish confession: "I went on vacation for a week and decided to see what would happen if I abandoned the diet. Well, everything came rushing back—the itching, the pain, all of it. Believe me, you've convinced me!" When I saw Dr. B. on a six-month follow-up visit, he was no longer taking any prednisone at all, had returned to his practice, and was entirely back to normal. With one exception, of course.

"I think this made me a much better therapist," Dr. B. confides. "Now, when I see patients in my practice referred by their doctors who tell them, 'Oh, it's all in your head,' I don't buy it for a minute—because that's just what my doctors told me. The fact is, it's easier to give someone a psychological label than to admit you can't help them. Believe me, I know how diet can affect emotions, because I lived through it."

I wish I could say that Dr. B. is an isolated case. He's not. Rarely a week goes by that I do not see at least one—and often several—patients who turn out, upon tests, to have PCC. In fact, I believe PCC may be the single most underreported of any of the phantom diseases. Reliable sources have estimated that *as many as 30 percent of all Americans* may have PCC. I find that figure simply staggering. That would mean that *seventy-two million Americans* may be suffering from the effects of PCC. Another recent book puts the figure at eighty million! If those numbers seem boggling, I tell patients to think of it in a much more down-to-earth way: Three out of ten people you see on the street harbor some hidden, dangerous PCC infections. That includes your friends, your family, your mate or lover . . . and yourself.

Some experts call such figures exaggerated. Very well, for the sake of argument, suppose we arbitrarily decide to cut the 30 percent figure in half—that gives thirty-six million—and, to be extra cautious, halve it again—eighteen million. So you see, even by the most conservative drawing and quartering of the numbers, PCC is an astoundingly common problem.

What is clear, and generally agreed upon, is that *Candidiasis* is a much more common problem among women than it is among men. That is due, in part, to the fact that the vagina is an ideal "growth culture" for yeast—warm, moist, with rich mucosal surfaces. Not only is the vagina especially vulnerable to yeast organisms brought in from the outside world, but its delicate chemical balance is easily disrupted by contraceptives, douches, and spermicides, creating an ideal stage for yeast growth. Finally, women's more complex hormonal regulatory systems are prey to imbalances that, in turn, can promote the growth of yeast organisms.

## A Phantom of Many Faces

The reason PCC can be such a devil to track down is because it can take so many forms. I have culled this list of possible symptoms from several popular books on the subject, as well as research papers. Have you noticed any of these?

| | |
|---|---|
| Fatigue | Psoriasis |
| Lethargy | Hyperactivity |
| Depression | Cramps and abdominal |
| Inability to concentrate | pain |
| Headaches | Diarrhea |
| Skin problems | Gas |
| Difficulty breathing | Bloating |
| Vaginitis | Coated tongue |
| Joint pain/swelling | Muscle cramps/aches |
| Vaginal burning or itching | Muscle weakness |
| Rectal pain or itching | Lowered sex drive |

If it seems like an unbelievably wide range of symptoms—no wonder—it is. In fact, it is this wide range of symptoms that has caused incredible disagreement about PCC. Before we get to what you need to know to track down this phantom in your life, let's look briefly at what the brouhaha is all about.

## Now You See It . . .

I would be less than candid if I did not tell you something of the extraordinary controversy surrounding this particular phantom. Several corners of the medical establishment—from the *Harvard Health Letter* to the American Academy of Allergy—have gone out of their way to deny that there is any such thing as PCC. They call it a fictitious disease. Again and again, they pooh-pooh suggestive findings and case histories, branding it a "fringe movement," a "fad," or worse.

At base, this medical attitude is curiously schizoid. When it comes to yeast infections, the medical establishment plays a fast and furious game of "now you see it, now you don't." On the one hand, even the most staid physicians have long recognized localized yeast infections. Gynecologists, cancer specialists, and pediatricians see them routinely: in women, transplant patients, AIDS patients, children, and immunocompromised patients. Yet, they insist, yeast does not spread into a more systemic infection. Those who seem to have such a disease, they say, must be wrong, malingering, or just plain neurotic.

Their argument would be more compelling if traditional practitioners could offer something to help such patients—but they can't. Again and again, orthodox medical science turns away such patients, unable to help them. Yet these same people find their way to me, to my colleagues, or to any of the practitioners now becoming aware of the tremendous discoveries around PCC, and then often show remarkable improvement. Not always, nor always completely—but enough so that it is clear something is going

## BODY PARTS AND SYSTEMS
## AFFECTED BY YEAST INFECTIONS

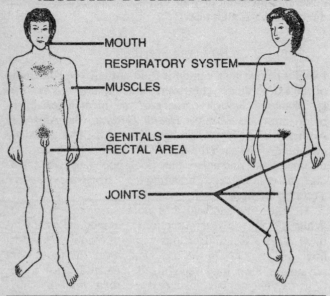

MOUTH

RESPIRATORY SYSTEM

MUSCLES

GENITALS
RECTAL AREA

JOINTS

on that seems beyond the reach of the conventional medical wisdom.

Penny was just such a case. For nine years she had been extremely ill. Her problem was as embarrassing as it was acute: She could not stray more than a few minutes from a toilet. Every day she was wracked with agonizing stomach spasms and gastrointestinal upset that would send her racing to the nearest lavatory. The problem had gotten so bad that for one entire year she was unable to leave her house. Her husband, Steve, did the shopping and took care of their two small children, and she could only watch as their happy family life disintegrated into a nightmare of illness and pain. Locked in what seemed to be a prison of her malady, she watched her children and her husband leading their own lives and cried that she could not share it with them.

Needless to say, she consulted doctors galore, but they found nothing. One sent her to a big-city specialist, who did nothing. Another sent her to a psychiatrist, who diagnosed "psychosomatic" illness and put her on antidepressants. Finally, she came to see me, where her lab tests showed a very different picture. Penny had an extreme reaction to yeast and eggs, so much so that eating even a single piece of bread could make her violently ill. Yet nobody, in all Penny's doctor visits, had thoroughly assessed her yeast intolerance. I put her on an appropriate diet, and today Penny has resumed her active, involved life with her family—with virtually no symptoms. Having seen such dramatic improvements, I cannot just write off the terrific successes of people like Penny and Dr. B.

But, in good conscience, I would like to review some of the arguments often marshaled against the phantom disease of PCC. After all, being an educated medical consumer means knowing both sides of the story. Besides, if you think you might be affected (more on how to tell that in the next few pages), you may well hear some of these arguments from the doctors you consult. I wouldn't be doing my job if I didn't tell you what people are saying—and what I think about their points—so you can draw your own conclusions.

## Note:

If you are more interested in how PCC may apply to your own situation and less interested in the medical pros and cons, I suggest you skip to the section "Let's Get Personal," on page 122.

## The "Too-Broad" Argument

The first argument you may hear against PCC is the one I mentioned above. Simply put, some critics say that the range of symptoms it can cause is too broad. It is simply not credible, say the critics, that one infection could cause so many diverse problems. Ergo, they say, it must be a fraud.

To be sure, the list of possible symptoms is staggering, as we have already seen, but I have two responses to this. First, we know of a number of diseases and infections that create a wide range of symptoms. In fact, there is no disease that always creates exactly the same narrow constellation of symptoms in every single person. Because the proposed mechanism of yeast infections involves systemic "poisoning" by yeast toxins, it doesn't seem surprising that symptoms can arise in whatever part of the body those toxins act on most strongly—be it your kidneys, brain, heart, liver, or muscles.

The second reason I don't buy that critique is simple: Just because PCC *can* manifest all those symptoms doesn't mean that it always does.

To dismiss it because the range of symptoms can be so broad seems both disingenuous and shortsighted. Yes, it can create a plethora of symptoms, but so can cancer and Parkinson's disease—but we don't dismiss them, do we?

## The "It Doesn't Make Sense" Argument

The next common argument goes like this: Because we can come up with no clear-cut, ready-made mechanism for why yeast infections cause the multitude of symptoms they do, therefore they must not really cause them.

If you ask me, this says more about the state of our medical understanding than it does about any biological truth. It is the same defense skeptics have used to "rebut" new advances ever since the germ theory: If we can't already explain it, it must not exist.

Yet by definition, new medical understanding happens when observed clinical problems go beyond what we already know—precisely what is happening with systemic *Candida* infections. As to the skeptics who refuse to believe it can cause such symptoms, I'd invite them to talk with some of the patients in my waiting room!

The easiest way to see the fallacy of this argument is simply to turn it around. If *Candida* is not the culprit, then what is? Can they explain why, after repeated visits to the best physicians, elaborate consultations, and extensive medical tests, patients can find nothing wrong? Until the Doubting Thomases can offer a better answer to that basic question, I think they owe their patients a second look at the yeast link.

## The "Unproven" Argument

This argument brands the yeast link as unproven and says that until the medical establishment has conducted its own large-scale, controlled studies, we cannot know if the symptoms attributed to yeast infections are in fact caused by them and whether the treatment actually helps.

Indeed, I know this argument well, because I used to believe it. When I first heard about PCC infections, I was quite a skeptic. After all, I had not heard PCC discussed in my medical-school classes at Tufts University, nor at Harvard University School of Public Health. Surely such prestigious pinnacles of scientific achievement would know about such a problem . . . right?

Apparently not. Today, after several years of seeing the differences such treatments have made in my own patients, I answer this differently: The proof is in the doing. There are patients who had something very seriously wrong, something no traditional medicine seemed to help. Today they are well. That has left me convinced that there is a profound, and underrecognized, medical truth at work here.

I recently appeared on a television show with four such PCC patients. These three women and a man had made progress that could only be termed spectacular. For a half hour they sat and described their symptoms, the devastation the diseases brought to their lives. They answered questions, telling candidly and bravely how their treatments had brought them back to sanity and health. Yet shortly after that performance, I chanced to meet a conservative medical colleague who still believes that yeast is all hoax and medical nonsense. I found myself wondering, with such sterling success stories available to examine, with hundreds of such cases repeated around the country, with such honest, courageous presentation by these patients, how long will it take until the medical establishment agrees to take a fair, honest look at the PCC problem? (It's times like that when being a doctor gets very frustrating!)

Is PCC fact or fiction? I can only point to my experience, and the experience of scores of patients and colleagues—and that says that it's a real problem. One can choose to believe it or not, but the fact is that every week I and my medical colleagues who treat yeast seriously see "miraculous" turn-arounds, helping people whose shattered lives are pieced back together again.

For my part, I cannot ignore it when patients get better. The fact is that when people get well—people for whom traditional medicine offers no answers and less hope—then there's clearly something worth at least exploring. So explore it we must. I am the first to agree that PCC has not been completely validated in the laboratory—not yet at least.

But while we're waiting for further breakthroughs from the laboratories, I keep coming back to one incontrovertible fact: I and the many other doctors working with PCC patients have watched this phantom validated time and again in the real-world "laboratories" of our own practice. So, in one way, I agree with this criticism. Let me be the first to agree that yes, there should be more studies and more research undertaken. I think it is high time the speculation was put to rest—and this phantom brought out of its closet once and for all.

## The Bottom Line: Yeast Doesn't Care

Now that we've gone through all the medical arguments, I want to remind you of just one thing. They are just that: arguments. Debates. But the brainless yeast beasties don't care one iota who wins those arguments. They couldn't care less whether we believe in them or not. For they are too busy doing their thing: multiplying and, I believe, making millions of us unhealthy.

So here is a disease from an organism doctors admit exists chronically in your body, whose presence shows up on laboratory antibody tests, which arguably causes immense physical and psychological problems, the elimination of which can bring dramatic reversals in sickness. Yet, most traditional doctors don't "believe" in it.

I hope you are starting to see a pattern here. A disease with elusive symptoms, physicians powerless to improve it, others branding it "all in your head," breathtaking cures transforming lives, and "experts" pooh-poohing them. If that combination starts to sound a bit familiar, it should—after all, it's the profile of a classic phantom disease.

## What *Do* the Scientists Say?

In spite of the fact that we still have much to learn about *Candida*, it seems that every month, some new study comes out adding another link to our understanding of this phantom. Following are a few representative tidings from the laboratory frontiers.

Chronic candidiasis may not be all in your head, but there's a strong possibility that it may manifest there. According to two reports in the *Journal of the American Medical Association,* one of the more insidious side effects of PCC may be depression. Scientists are just beginning to understand why this should be so, but it has been suggested by some physicians that a toxin produced by the yeast organism—known as canditoxin—can have significant effects on several of the body's biochemical systems. Physicians have reported the effect of this chemical on hormones, immune-system regulators, and even the chemical messengers, called neurotransmitters, that carry signals in the brain itself.

As we elucidate this biochemical brain link further, it may hold the key to several of the psychological symptoms that have been reported by PCC sufferers: anxiety, lethargy, nervousness, forgetfulness, and general mental confusion. We can also hope it will result in fewer people being tagged as "neurotic" and more of them getting the help they need for the true cause of their problems: the *Candida* organism.

## The Yeast-Immune Link

There is another very important area where yeast plays a role in your health and that is in your immune system. But the relationship is both complex and little understood. Simply put, *Candida* infections can be both a cause and an effect of subnormal immune function.

The cycle begins when the immune system is at a low ebb, which can occur for a variety of reasons: poor nutrition, excess stress, hidden cancer, any of several immunosuppressive conditions (including ARC and AIDS), too much exposure to sunlight, or taking immune-suppressing drugs, such as cortisone or other steroids.

When that happens, the usual immune factors that help keep yeast in check no longer do so, and the yeast colonies begin to proliferate. This begins a vicious cycle, for as they grow, they release chemical toxins that in *themselves* appear to weaken immune cells further. The result is an endless, vicious cycle of yeast-immune antagonism: more yeasts, more toxins, more immune damage. In this cellular tug-of-war, there is only one loser: you.

Clear support for the yeast-immune link is coming from research laboratories all over. One recent and provocative study involved women with chronic vaginal yeast problems. Researchers at Cornell Medical Center studied these womens' immune systems and found that fully three-quarters of them are unable to mount an adequate immune defense against the yeast organisms. In effect, their immune-system fails to recognize the fungus and so allows it to overrun the body's defenses to the point of a frank infection.

Obviously, it doesn't take much to realize that if your immune sentries can't fight yeast in the vagina, they also can't fight it elsewhere in the bloodstream or body. That means that the stage is set for ongoing, chronic *Candida* infections—and those staggering numbers, those millions of PCC victims, begin to make sense.

The immune-yeast link has been frequently noted with the grave immune disorder AIDS. It is now recognized that one of the signs of that disease can be the growth of yeast patches in the mouth and esophagus. It is often one of the first clinically observable manifestations of the disease. But you don't have to have AIDS to have those patches. Your grandmother knew that when you suffer from a cold or flu, which can temporarily depress your immune function, you may get the familiar "coated tongue." It's usually not serious, but simply a temporary, local overgrowth of yeast in the mouth—a rough and ready barometer of your current immune status.

From AIDS to the common cold, researchers and clinical physicians have seen quite clearly that yeast has intimate links with your immune system. But we are now learning that it also seems to be associated with many other diseases. One study, from Johns Hopkins Hospital, found that almost three out of four people with chronic *Candidiasis*—70 percent—also had some serious associated disease. The diseases included pernicious anemia, cirrhosis, and diseases of glandular systems including thyroid, parathyroid, and adrenal glands. Other studies have shown links to myasthenia gravis and the skin conditions psoriasis and vitiligo.

Which comes first—these manifold other problems or the *Candida* infections—is unclear. But it suggests again that PCC is a disease of a fundamental imbalance, which can affect hormones, immune function, and a range of the body's systems.

## Let's Get Personal

By now I think it is plenty clear that I am a "true believer" in this phantom, both because of the published research and because of my own clinical experience. I have seen it at work, not only in the devastating effects it can take on people's health and vitality but in the dramatic transformations that come about when people take appropriate anti-*Candida* measures.

So what I want to do now is to leave the abstract arguments behind and talk about you:

• What *you* need to know about PCC
• How its symptoms may affect *your* life
• How to know if *you* have the signs
• What *you* can do about it if you do

Enough now, with the "you"-seless debate. Let's look at the information from the only point of view that counts: yours.

## What Are Your Chances?

Usually, the first question people ask me is just who has problems with *Candida*. Is there some common factor, some Achilles' heel that puts us at risk? The answer is: absolutely. Do you fit into any of these categories?

### *Candida* Risk Profile

1. Do you take oral contraceptives? ___
2. Are you pregnant? ___
3. Have you had several pregnancies? ___
4. Are you taking, now or in the last year, antibiotics (see list on page 125) ___
5. Do you take cortisone, prednisone, or other immunosuppressive drugs? ___
6. Are you undergoing chemotherapy? ___
7. Do you have chronic athlete's foot, "jock itch," or fingernail infections? ___
8. Has your doctor suggested that you may be immune-suppressed? ___
9. Have you had surgery recently? ___
10. Have you been under unusual stress? ___

There are other factors that have been implicated in PCC, but these are some of the most common. If you feel you can fit into these categories, there is at least a chance that you may be one of the millions of people at risk for PCC.

## The Antibiotic-*Candida* Link

*"The quickest way to get some sort of a yeast problem is to take a lot of antibiotics; you can experience symptoms within days of doing so."*

—Sidney Baker, M.D.
Gesell Institute of Child Development
New Haven, Connecticut

Undoubtedly the most common reason people get PCC is because of our society's profligate use of antibiotics. Widespread *Candida* infections were rarely observed in the days before antibiotics were so widely prescribed. But now, physicians prescribe an immense number of what are termed wide-spectrum antibiotics. These drugs live up to their name, because they kill a wide spectrum of organisms in the body. Often, they are given when doctors don't know exactly what the problem is but know that there is some infection at work.

These drugs are the pharmacological equivalent of thermonuclear bombs—they kill most everything in their path. Unfortunately, the organisms they kill are often the ones that are policing the yeast colonies. Once these microbial "enforcers" are killed, yeast can then proliferate in the intestinal or genitourinary tract, setting the stage for more widespread, systemic infection. It is a perfect example of how overenthusiastic doctoring creates a chain reaction of phantom, iatrogenic illness—and of how you can be the victim.

The fact is you are exposed to these antibiotics in a number of ways. If you have been hospitalized or operated on, you very likely received a dose. If you are one of the people who has taken a prolonged course of antibiotics for acne, it is certain that the balance of organisms in your digestive tract has been altered. Likewise, if you have taken massive antibiotics for any sort of infection in the last year, you might be at PCC risk.

You may want to get up right now and take a quick

guided tour of your medicine cabinet. Does it contain any of the widely prescribed antibiotics that can disturb your *Candida* balance?

| | |
|---|---|
| Achromycin | Keflex |
| Amoxicillin | Minocin |
| Ampicillin | Panmycin |
| Anspor | Retet |
| Azo Gantanol | SAS-500 |
| Azulfidine | Septra |
| Bactrim | Sumycin |
| Ceclor | Tetraclor |
| Cephalosporin | Tetracycline |
| Ceporex | Tetracyn |
| Cyclopar | Tetram |
| Gantanol | Vibramycin |

## Yeast and the Pill

Women who take oral contraceptives are also at higher risk for PCC problems, according to several studies. This is because oral contraceptives disturb the usual hormonal and biochemical balance in your body. Once that equilibrium has been disturbed, yeast organisms can take over. I recently ran across a paper in a British medical journal that mentioned two very interesting correlations:

• Before the introduction of the Pill, the incidence of *Candida* infection was virtually nil.
• When the Pill was introduced, there was a corresponding rise in the rate of *Candida* infections.

Today, the physicians noted, approximately four women out of ten they see in their gynecological practice report problems with yeast infections each year. In this country, vaginal yeast infections—not the same as PCC, but certainly a related condition indicating an immune imbalance in the body's defenses against yeast—occur in one-quarter of women who visit gynecologists. It is not clear how many of these are directly due to oral contraceptives, but it is quite certain that their use makes it more likely that you will suffer from localized—and perhaps systemic—yeast infections.

## You Are What You Eat . . .

Finally, there is a more insidious, and common, way you may receive a significant dose of antibiotics. Most of the meat and poultry raised commercially—and food that finds its way to your dinner plate—is chock full of antibiotics in the commercial feed lots. These drugs help deliver a plump, juicy steak or chicken to your dinner table, and the food producers a juicier bottom line, but the hidden drugs they carry take their toll on your body by delivering a constant low-level bombardment of steroids, additives, and antibiotics.

Whether they come from your medicine chest or your dinner table, the antibiotics you ingest can tip your biological scale in the direction of chronic candidiasis infection.

## Give Yourself a PCC Check

Like the causes behind them, the symptoms of this disease are extraordinarily diverse. In this, they show the hallmark of most phantom diseases. Armed with what you know from the above, here is a list of the more common PCC symptoms. I suggest that you take a moment and check yourself against it. This list was developed by Seroyal Laboratories, a leading *Candida*-treatment manufacturer.

## A Note on Test Taking

Because there are so many symptoms, and they are so broad-ranging, you should not be concerned if you show a few of them. Given the general state of dis-ease present in our population—thanks to our medical sickness-based model—it's very possible that you may "register" on one or more variables. But what you should be alert to are patterns, constellations of symptoms clustered together that suggest a possible PCC link. Psychiatrists call this a gestalt. I call it good, solid diagnostic detective work. Don't worry if you have only a few sporadic, possible signs. What counts is a clear pattern.

When I have explained this to patients, they often ask, "How do I know whether I really have the symptoms or am just thinking I might?"

My answer is to paraphrase jazz great Duke Ellington, who said, "If you have to ask, you don't have it." Before you decide you have a given symptom, you should pass the "reasonable-observer test." Ask yourself, "Is this so clear and definite that any reasonable observer would agree that I suffer from this problem?" If you can answer yes objectively, go ahead and count it. If not, don't.

| | |
|---|---|
| Fatigue | Rectal pain or itching |
| Lethargy | Poor coordination |
| Depression | Psoriasis |
| Inability to concentrate, feeling "spacy" or "disconnected" | Hyperactivity |
| | Cramps and abdominal pain |
| | Diarrhea |
| Headaches | Gas |
| Skin problems | Bloating |
| Difficulty breathing | Coated tongue |
| Vaginitis | Muscle cramps/aches |
| Joint pain/swelling | Muscle weakness |
| Vaginal burning, itching, or discharge | Lowered sex drive |
| | Severe bad breath |

## Do You See Yourself Here?

If, on the basis of this inventory, you feel you may be one of those suffering from an undiagnosed PCC condition, there are two avenues open to you. Or, more accurately, they are like two sides to the same coin of *Candida* health: doctors and diet. Let's take a quick look at the first: getting appropriate help.

Obviously, in order to get help with a phantom *Candida* condition, you need a physician who understands the complexities of this syndrome. When you are feeling sick, fatigued, or depressed—the hallmarks of *Candida*—the last thing you need is to fight with your doctor to persuade him or her that it's not all in your head. You may have a perfectly wonderful, open-minded, and informed personal physician, one who is either informed about the newest PCC research or is willing to learn.

But if not, or if you feel you want to go to a specialist in this area, I include the ''For Deeper Study'' section, at the end of this chapter, which suggests resources where you can get a listing of a yeast-aware physician near you.

To track down the phantom, your doctor will do two things: First, he or she will take a very detailed medical and life-style history, similar to the profile you have already filled out in this chapter. The next step will be some tests. Your doctor may first order a stool culture, the traditional test for *Candida* overgrowth. The idea is that if your digestive tract is overrun with yeasts, it will show up in your body's waste product. However, there is some concern that this doesn't always pinpoint the problem.

Others may move directly to a series of blood tests. There is extraordinary debate raging about how useful these tests are. The real problem is that since all of us have yeast in our bodies all the time, we all have antibodies to them as well. Obviously, that makes culturing yeast or measuring yeast antibodies fairly imprecise.

However, research has shown that a combination of tests

may prove the most useful. By running three tests, medical researchers found they could derive a reasonably certain diagnosis. In case you want to discuss the matter with your doctor, the tests are

- Enzyme immunoassay (ELISA) test for *Candida* antigen (CAg)
- Enzyme immunoassay (ELISA) test for *Candida* antibody (CAb)
- Counter-immuno electrophoresis test for *Candida* antibody (CIE CAb)

Taken together, this three-test series has given a positive predictive value of 100 percent for people with true systemic *Candida* infections.

While the technical specifications seem complex, they boil down to a hopeful bottom line: We are learning how to make much more accurate, sensitive, and reliable diagnoses of *Candida* infections.

The final thing your doctor will probably do, if your condition warrants it, is to give you an antiyeast antibiotic. At this point, I hope you let out a resounding "What?!?" If you've been following along, you probably wonder why—after all, isn't it antibiotics that help cause *Candida* overgrowth in the first place? How can taking more of them help you?

While this may sound like the medical equivalent of the "hair of the dog that bit you" cure, there is a real logic to it. Remember that I said that the antibiotics that cause the problems in the first place are like nuclear bombs. Well, the drug used to fight the yeast beast is instead a guided missile. The drug, called Nystatin, zeros in primarily on the yeasts in your digestive tract. It does very little else because it is barely absorbed into your body at all—most of it is excreted. That means that it kills the yeast at their source—in your bowels—but leaves you otherwise largely untouched. For this reason, the drug has virtually no side effects and is considered the treatment of choice for confirmed *Candida* infections.

## Patient, Heal Thyself

Of course, by far the best medicine is no medicine at all, and for many *Candida* patients, there is a course of "treatments" that actually work without taking anything at all. They involve making some careful and consistent dietary changes.

For some people, just making these changes in what they eat, drink, and ingest may be enough to tip the scales back, reducing your body's load of hitchhiking yeasts and letting your own immune defenses rid your body of the problem. For others, dietary measures are most effective when used in conjunction with an initial Nystatin treatment. But whichever of these courses you take, diet is an absolutely vital factor in getting and staying free from yeast invaders.

There are several sources describing excellent antiyeast diets, which you will find in the resources section at the end of this chapter. All of these diets, however, boil down to three basic principles in the yeast battle.

## Step One: Cut Their Supply Lines!

If this is a war, you should conduct yourself like a general. So, if the problem is too many yeast troops taking over your body, the last thing you want to do is send them reinforcements, right? That means that your first step is to close the door against further yeast overgrowth, by *removing yeasts, as much as possible, from everything you eat*.

It seems obvious. By eliminating yeast organisms from the food and drink you take in, you stop adding to the yeast load your body has to cope with. As you stop overloading your body's defenses, you give nature's own mechanisms the chance to come back into healthy equilibrium.

Not surprisingly, this is more easily said than done. Obviously, none of us sit down to consume cakes or packets of yeast. (Believe me, if you tried it, you'd never do it again!) But the fact is that we don't need to, for these tiny organisms are stealthy, furtive invaders. Like the Trojan soldiers in their famous wooden horse, yeasts slip into your body by hiding in nutritious food and drink. Your best defense, then, is knowing where they may be coming in, and which are the prime yeast-containing foods, so that you can stop this flood of new yeast invaders *before* they take up residence in your body.

Take a look at this list of common, everyday foods. Can you identify which one are the prime "Yeast Danger" foods?

| | | | |
|---|---|---|---|
| Cookies | —— | Sour cream | —— |
| Cakes | —— | Mushrooms | —— |
| Whole wheat bread | —— | Sauerkraut | —— |
| Cinnamon rolls | —— | Fruit juices | |
| Pickles | —— | (bottled, frozen, canned) | —— |
| Vinegar | —— | Dried fruit | —— |
| Pickle relish | —— | Melons | —— |
| Mustard | —— | Buttermilk | —— |
| Ketchup | —— | Crème fraîche | —— |
| Cheese | —— | Coq au vin | —— |
| Barbecue chips | —— | Green olives | —— |
| Smoked meats | —— | Bottled salad dressings | —— |
| "Dry-roasted" nuts | —— | Canned soups | —— |
| Tamari sauce | —— | Soy sauce | —— |
| Pickled herring | —— | Alcohol cocktails | —— |

Ready for the answer? Well, I admit—it was a trick question. *Every one* of the foods listed here contains yeast, fungus, or spores that can exacerbate *Candidiasis* conditions. But these are only the worst of the problem-causing foods. The complete list could go on for page after page! (If you are interested, the "For Deeper Study" section suggests several resources that offer complete lists of yeast-danger foods.) Now that you know the truth, I suggest you go back through the list again, but this time, mark only those that you have eaten in the past week. If you're like most people, you'll find an alarmingly heavy dose of hidden "Trojan horse" yeasts.

## Step Two: Starve Them Out

You've already seen that step one means closing the door, eliminating the introduction of more yeast into your system. Now you are ready for the next phase: starving them out.

By making appropriate dietary changes, you can deny the *Candida* colonies in your digestive tract the nutrients they need. By putting these yeast beasts on an "elimination diet," it is thought that you can greatly reduce their flourishing growth in your gut. The fewer of them there are, the lower the risk that they will proliferate out of control, sending *Candida* toxins throughout your body.

Yeasts have simple tastes: sugar, sugar, and more sugar. (That's why Aunt Mabel's bread recipes always start with "Dissolve sugar and yeast in warm water.") It follows that if you eat a lot of sweets, particularly refined, high-potency sugars, you are feeding the yeasts exactly what they need.

Clearly, if sugars were the only culprit, it would be easy to deal with—simply cut them out. But yeasts are more clever, and more versatile, than that. What they really love is carbohydrates—from pizza and pasta to breads and rolls. It makes sense, because carbohydrates are broken down into sugars in your body, so yeasts are ideal secondary sources of the basic sugar the yeast thrives on. Needless to say, when you mix the two, in sweet carbohydrates—the cakes, cookies, rolls, and breads that are so irresistible—you are providing an ideal diet for your yeast invaders (nothing could make your yeast organisms happier!). With our diets high in these elements, no wonder our nation has such an out-of-control yeast problem.

While these two kinds of foods encourage yeast growth similarly, the nutritional prescription for them is not the same. For the sticky-sweet desserts, the answer is fairly simple: Just say no. That's a good idea for several reasons. Not only do these sweets provide fuel for your unwanted yeast colonies, they also provide destructive, empty calories that become unsightly, unhealthy fat and that create wild "sugar rush" swings of mood, energy, and emotion. Of these, the less said—and the less eaten—the better.

If you worry that that may be a hardship, consider the following study, from the *Journal of Reproductive Medicine.* A physician team reported on one hundred women with chronic *Candida* infections. When the women drastically reduced their intake of sucrose, dairy products containing milk sugars, and artificial sweeteners, they had a marked drop in severity and frequency of their *Candida* problems. The report termed the difference "dramatic." For most PCC sufferers, being able to feel a "dramatic" change in their health is more than worth a few cookies and cakes! So much for sugars.

Carbohydrates, on the other hand, present a more complex story. As I pointed out at length in my last book, *How to Be Your Own Nutritionist,* for most of us, making carbohydrates the centerpiece of your diet is good nutrition. In proper amounts and variety, these "starches" help reduce fats, cancer, minimize energy swings, and increase the amount of healthy fiber you take in.

Yet for people with severe chronic yeast problems, these carbos are a mixed blessing. For such patients, I recommend a high-protein, low-fat diet during the yeast-reduction phases. That allows you to clear out the excess yeast overload, without working against yourself as you do so.

Then, when your *Candida* situation has returned to a healthy and stable norm and your symptoms have abated, you can gradually, and gently, begin reintroducing carbohydrates—in reasonable quantity.

Here, as a sample, is what such a yeast-elimination diet would look like:

## *Candida* Diet Menus

**Day One:**

*Breakfast:*
Ground beef patty
Whole wheat yeast-free cracker
Grapefruit

*Lunch:*
Tuna salad on bed of lettuce
Rice cakes
Steamed green beans almondine
Strawberries

*Dinner:*
Broiled lamb chops
Steamed broccoli and cauliflower
Baked potato with chives
Nectarine

**Day Two:**

*Breakfast:*
Oatmeal
Berries
Almonds

*Lunch:*
  Sliced turkey breast
  Carrot and celery sticks
  Yeast-free crackers
  Apple

*Dinner:*
  Broiled fish
  Steamed wax beans
  Wild rice with cashews and vegetables
  Kiwi

## Day Three:

*Breakfast:*
  Poached eggs
  Sautéed potato
  Fresh pineapple

*Lunch:*
  Three-bean salad with oil, lemon and onion
  Chilled steamed broccoli
  Pear

*Dinner:*
  Tossed green salad
  Lean steak
  Baked acorn squash
  Broiled tomato
  Peach

## Day Four:

*Breakfast:*
  Rice cakes with cashew butter
  Sliced banana

*Lunch:*
   Pork chop
   Boiled cabbage
   Unsweetened applesauce

*Dinner:*
   Baked Cornish hen
   Barley pilaf
   Steamed asparagus
   Grapes

## Day Five:

*Breakfast:*
   Barley cereal
   Strawberries
   Pecans

*Lunch:*
   Spinach salad with egg
   Pine nuts
   Orange

*Dinner:*
   Tossed green salad
   Lemon chicken with snow peas
   Steamed baby carrots or baked potato

## Beverages:

   Seltzer
   Mineral water
   Water

## Dressings:

   Lemon juice
   Vegetable oils
   Garlic
   Onions
   Herbs

Dr. Jeffrey Bland, biochemist at the Linus Pauling Institute, has suggested another dietary weapon you can use to help fight *Candida* overgrowth. Bland found that giving patients an oral supplement of *Lactobacillus acidophilus,* one teaspoon three times a day, helps reestablish the natural balance of microorganisms, the intestinal flora that your body wants. You'll recall that it is the disturbance of these organisms—by antibiotics or other factors—that often unleashes *Candida* problems in the first place. Bland's use of *acidophilus* bacteria seems to help put things back in balance, and he reports encouraging successes with *Candida* patients. He has also tried linking this treatment with supplements of the B vitamin biotin, which seems to hamper yeast's transformation into its invasive, mycelial form.

## Step Three: Remember Your Vitamins and Minerals!

The third front of the yeast battle involves micronutrients, that is, vitamins and minerals. There is a good deal of research showing that people with PCC infections have imbalances of several crucial nutrients:

- A study from London shows that three-quarters of the sample of chronic *Candidiasis* patients studied showed evidence of iron deficiency, with low levels of iron in their blood and low iron stores.
- From the Gesell Institute, in New Haven, a study shows that a sample of patients with abnormally low levels of the crucial micronutrient magnesium had an abnormally high sensitivity to *Candida*-reaction tests. Other scientists report that "magnesium deficiency is the single most common nutritional deficiency among patients with *Candidiasis.*"
- A study in the *Journal of Infectious Diseases* found that among a group of patients with local yeast infections, more than half had levels of vitamin A and beta-

carotene below minimum levels. In fact, even among people whose levels were above the cut-off point, *all* of them had levels in the lowest half of the measurement range.

In 1986, researchers in Scotland found that a deficiency of the mineral selenium weakens the immune response to *Candida albicans* in *in vitro* laboratory tests.

There is much more research implicating specific nutrients in patients with chronic or severe yeast infections, and more is coming out every month. While there is much we still have to learn, what is already quite clear is that a balance of essential nutrients is extremely important in keeping the yeast beast at bay.

I believe these nutrients work in two ways: first, by direct action on the *Candida* organisms themselves, and second, by strengthening your overall immune health, so that your body's own immune gatekeepers can do a better job of keeping yeast from growing out of control.

## The Last Word

I don't usually indulge in predictions, but in this case, I will break that rule. It is my belief that the next two years will bring a breathtaking boom in our understanding of yeast infections—their causes, detection, and treatment. I certainly hope so, because it is high time we bring this phantom out into the light and expose it to thorough medical scrutiny.

If this chapter has raised more questions for you than it has answered, that's fine. The area of yeast infections is so new, so controversial, and so inadequately understood that I hope you will be interested in exploring it further. Here is a short, annotated bibliography of some of what I consider to be the best resources to help you do that. Good luck!

## For Deeper Study

C. Orian Truss, M.D., *The Missing Diagnosis*. P.O. Box 26508, Birmingham, Alabama 35226. The classic book on the subject, by the discoverer of PCC.

John Parks Trowbridge, M.D., and Morton Walker, D.P.M., *The Yeast Syndrome*. New York: Bantam Books, 1986. The single most up-to-date book, including a list of yeast-aware physicians.

William G. Crook, M.D., *The Yeast Connection*. New York: Vintage Books, 1985. A broad, authoritative source book for lay readers.

Leo Galland, M.D. "Nutrition and *Candida Albicans*." In *A Year in Nutritional Medicine,* ed. Jeffrey Bland, Ph.D., New Canaan, Conn.: Keats Publishing Corp., 1986.

# 8

# The Fatal Phantom: Silent Ischemia

When it comes to phantom diseases, you have already seen some of the many ways they can be terribly destructive. We have witnessed the toll they take on the quality of life, sapping your energy and vigor, depleting your reserves, dulling your mind, and distorting your emotions. If this alone were the extent of the phantoms' damage, they would still represent a tremendously serious public health problem. Unfortunately, they reach well beyond this.

For as difficult as these illnesses may be to deal with, all of them have one thing in common. While intensely destructive, the phantoms we have discussed until now are rarely deadly. Their importance comes from the serious, chronic health problems they create and the cumulative load they place on our nation's health.

Now, in these next two chapters, we will explore two phantom diseases with a more serious side. They both involve your cardiovascular system—the heart and blood vessels. Like all true phantoms, they are little recognized and even more rarely diagnosed. But these two phantoms can do more than cripple; if allowed to sneak up on us, they can even kill. What's more, we know as a medical and statistical fact that both these phantoms touch the lives of many millions of Americans—people who don't even have the faintest suspicion that anything is wrong. Yet as widespread as they are, these phantoms manage to remain in the medical closet.

## Public Enemy Number One—Silent Ischemia

When it comes to the first of these, I will be very surprised if you have even heard of it. It goes by several names, but nowadays is most commonly known as silent myocardial ischemia—SMI, for short.

Beneath that complex medical name is really a rather simple condition. First, let's dispense with the Latin. *Myocardial* refers to the heart muscle, and *ischemia* means "lacking in adequate oxygen." Together, they make a dangerous combination. But ironically, the worst aspect of this phantom comes not from those three-dollar words, but from the part of its name that you understood right away: *silent*.

The hallmark of this phantom is that it can strike without warning, without any telltale signs to announce itself. Invisible and painless, it can do its biological damage without its victims ever knowing anything was amiss.

The words of one recent medical paper put it bluntly: "Sudden cardiac death may be the only clinical sign in asymptomatic patients." I admit, I can think of nothing more disturbing than a disease where your first symptom is also your last. That's the bad news.

But there is good news here, too—lest you be too worried. Happily, SMI can be relatively easy to diagnose and treat—if you and your doctor know just how and when to look for it. My pledge to you is that after reading this chapter, you will.

## What's in a Name?

As its name implies, ischemia is a condition in which your heart temporarily doesn't get enough oxygen-rich blood. In that respect, it is close cousin to what happens in an attack of *angina pectoris* or even a heart attack (myocardial infarction). The crucial difference is that, for reasons we do not understand very well, SMI doesn't give you the signals those other conditions do. As T. S. Eliot might have said, this is a disease that creeps on little cat's feet, silent and stealthy.

One way it can move undetected is that the factors that create SMI build up gradually. The long road to ischemia is the same one we have all heard about over and over again for heart disease.

When fatty plaque deposits settle in the coronary arteries supplying blood to your heart, their walls thicken. As the hollow part of the artery (what doctors call the lumen) shrinks, its capacity to deliver blood gradually drops. Biologically, it is the precise equivalent of a sludged up, partially blocked plumbing line.

During this gradual process, the heart is often not damaged severely. But then, without warning, one of two things may happen. For one of several reasons, the artery may have a spasm. Then, like a fist closing, the muscle-lined artery wall contracts, closing off the already thickened artery. Blood may be totally cut off or reduced so far that the heart cannot function normally.

The same thing can happen if your blood has a free-floating blood clot. As it tries to pass through, it gets stuck in the narrowed artery, blocking blood flow, with the same result.

The reason that this is a phantom disease is that, unlike classic angina, you feel no sharp pain, no shortness of breath. Unlike a classic heart attack, you feel no constricting tightness of the chest, no discomfort radiating into your arms. In fact, you feel nothing at all, which is what makes it so particularly worrisome.

There are unknown factors in the physiology of SMI that seem to short-circuit Nature's own built-in alarm mechanism. As a result, you feel none of the overt symptoms that usually accompany heart oxygen starvation. Medical experts still do not know how or why silent ischemia works this way, or why some people feel nothing in a situation where others feel intense pain. In fact, scientists are currently studying this mechanism intensively to try to solve the riddle.

There is yet another way in which this phantom creeps up on you. Most heart conditions manifest during strenuous exercise or acute periods of stress. It makes sense—after all, that's when your body places its fullest strain on your heart. But this quiet phantom happens in quiet moments, usually not at peaks of physical activity but at peaks of mental activity or at random times during ordinary daily activities. Two studies show that SMI episodes occur most often during such relatively normal activities as driving a car, reading, public speaking, and being interviewed.

But although this phantom may come with minimal signs, it can cause maximal damage. For when the heart muscle is deprived of normal blood flow, significant portions of the vital muscle become starved for oxygen. Then, in what is termed *ischemia necrosis,* the oxygen-starved heart cells can wither and die.

This is what a strong, normal heartbeat looks like on an electrocardiogram:

ECG tracing of normal heart rhythms

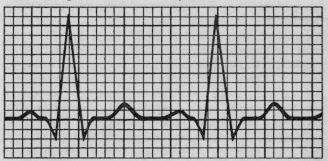

Compare what happens during a silent ischemic attack (see page 144).

When this happens in a heart attack or an episode of angina, we are immediately alarmed and do something about it—get to a hospital, take medications, see a physician. But with silent ischemia, we may not.

ECG tracing of ischemic heart rhythms

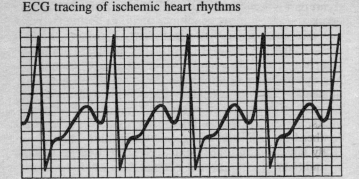

That means that one such subtle episode may only start off a vicious cycle. People with SMI often have attacks on a regular basis as they go about their daily lives—driving a car, working at a desk, even lying down. In fact, research indicates that such silent episodes appear to happen more often, and last longer, than painful heart attacks. Of course, with each silent attack, some part of their heart can become disabled, weakening the muscle and opening the door to other heart problems.

Little by little, this silent predator can erode a strong heart, leaving a person quite literally "faint-hearted." Ultimately, if a critical mass of the heart has been damaged, any one of these ischemic episodes can become the last. Nibbled away piece by piece, the heart may be pushed over the biological brink. Then the hapless victim can suffer either a full-blown classic heart attack or sudden cardiac death.

## The Deadly, Silent Quarter

We are just beginning to glimpse how frequently this phantom strikes. One recent study, in the *American Journal of Medicine,* revealed that one in four people who died suddenly of heart failure never had reported any symptoms whatsoever, yet were found on autopsy to have had chronic heart damage, the telltale sign of the ischemic phantom at work.

Other research indicates that the exact same percentage—25 percent—of heart attacks seem to happen without people being aware of them, indeed, without even knowing that their heart has been damaged. A recent follow-up to the landmark Framingham heart study found that, of more than seven hundred people who suffered heart attacks, 30 percent of the attacks were silent, recognized neither by the people not by their doctors.

By now, the truth behind this "deadly quarter" should be quite clear: They are the victims of this silent, stalking phantom of ischemia.

## Old Illness, New Discoveries

It would be hard to imagine a problem where the need to unmask it was so urgent. The good news here is that we are making great progress against it. This silent syndrome was first suggested about half a century ago, but until very recently it received virtually no public attention. In recent years, however, research developments have allowed us to diagnose and identify people with the problem reliably and accurately and thus treat them with an arsenal of cardiac drugs. One sign of our increased awareness of the problem occurred at a recent annual national scientific meeting of the American Heart Association, where several teams of researchers and scientists presented a comprehensive spectrum of new findings:

- Between four and five million people in this country are estimated to be endangered by silent ischemia.
- Even though it creates no symptoms, other studies show that this disease may strike from 2.5 to 10 percent of the population.
- This phantom is directly responsible for several tens of thousands of deaths annually, but contributes indirectly to many more.

When I first explain this to my patients, I know it can sound very frightening. But what I tell them next is that there is definitely a silver lining to this cloud. Because, for the first time, this research blitz is giving us a new and invaluable window on the workings and habits of this phantom. In recent years, cutting-edge research has given us powerful tools to detect, track down, predict, and treat people with SMI. Yes, we know more than ever before about the grim toll this phantom takes, but this same new effort has also taught us more than we ever knew about what to do to stop the disease *before* it takes its silent toll—so that it never will.

## It's Up to You

The very fact that so much of this is new knowledge gives *you* an especially important role to play. Many physicians, educated before our new and growing awareness of SMI, may not have gotten adequate training on the subject in their classes in medical school. In fact, according to Dr. Peter Cohn, a nationally recognized expert on SMI and chief of cardiology at the Health Sciences Center at Stony Brook, New York, "There is still a school of thought that believes 'No pain, no worry.' " Indeed, that is the old-line medical wisdom on this disease, an understanding that is fast being eclipsed by our new scientific understanding.

That suggests to me that there is all the more reason you should know the latest findings now. Because so much of this research is quite recent—it almost certainly has occurred since your doctor finished his or her formal medical training—it is doubly important that you do your part to be well informed.

I recently read an abstract by one of the premier researchers in this field. He concluded it with these words: "Silent myocardial ischemia is an important public health issue." Until the medical establishment wakes up to this fact and does a better job of incorporating it into our patient education, it's up to you to make sure it doesn't become a personal health issue for you or your loved ones.

## Check Your Own Risk

The first place to start is by looking at the risk profile below. If you see yourself here, it is especially vital that you take an active role in discussing the possibility of SMI with the physician you trust. Corny as it may sound, the life you save may be your own—or that of someone you love.

## Whom Does This Phantom Pick On?

With silent ischemia, as with much coronary disease, there is a relatively clear-cut hierarchy of those at risk. That's the place to start your own "self-exam" for this phantom. Do any of these describe you?

### SMI Risk Profile

| | |
|---|---|
| I am a diabetic | — |
| I am a smoker | — |
| I have high cholesterol | — |
| I have high blood pressure (hypertension) | — |
| My family has a history of heart disease | — |
| I have had one or more heart attacks | — |
| I have been diagnosed with angina | — |
| I have occasional sharp chest pains | — |

If the answer to any one of these is yes, you may well be at risk for SMI. But before you get too worried, remember, I said "at risk." That is *in no way* a diagnosis. *It doesn't mean you have it.* Not even close. Instead, you should view it as a lucky opportunity, because you are one of the fortunate ones. You have the chance to take steps *now* to lessen the risk of becoming a sorry "silent statistic."

That's exactly what I told Kent, one of my patients. On the face of it, Kent is exactly the sort of person that doctors usually dismiss with a reassuring "you're healthy as a horse." To be sure, on cursory examination, he was. Forty-four years old, the father of three children, Kent was making a handsome living as a financial analyst for a nationwide entertainment conglomerate. He had come to see me for what he called "my fifty-thousand-mile check"— not because anything was particularly wrong, but because he wanted to keep it that way.

Most of Ken's exam checked out fine, with the exception of slightly high blood pressure and cholesterol. Neither were, in and of themselves, alarming. I have no doubt that many more traditionally oriented physicians would have sent him away with the standard cautionary stories, exhorted him to "watch it," and left it at that. But two things tipped off my intuition. First, he mentioned in passing that he got more easily winded climbing stairs than he used to. "It's not a big thing, doc. Just getting old, I guess!" The other fact: that his father had suffered a major coronary at age fifty-two—and died nine years later from heart problems.

Neither fact by itself, but the juxtaposition of these several factors, told me Kent was a prime candidate for SMI. As I explained this, he was highly skeptical. "But how can there be something wrong with my ticker? I feel perfectly fine." I told him that I thought he *was* perfectly fine, but why not make absolutely sure? He agreed, and I sent him to a specialized cardiac clinic, with instructions for a specific SMI diagnostic test.

Ten days later he was back, with a new note of concern in his voice. The state-of-the-art electronics of the test revealed that his heart was already showing the beat pattern characteristic of early-stage SMI. It strongly suggested that his heart had already suffered hidden SMI damage and that Kent had some significant early problems developing in his coronary arteries.

With Kent, as with so many people, this story has a

happy ending. Armed with that information, I put Kent on a tightly controlled regime of diet, exercise, micronutrient supplementation, and drug therapy. Not only would it help rebuild his heart strength, it would also help clean out his blocked arteries and arrest further deterioration. He would have, in the most literal sense, a true "change of heart"— one that could save his life.

While I cannot promise that Kent is now completely off the danger list, I know that his odds are far better. Together we were able to nip in the bud his SMI condition that, had it continued unchecked, could very likely have spelled medical disaster for Kent and his family in a few years. The value of such preemptive medical sleuthing is that it lets us track down a cardiac killer before it hits— while we still have time to turn it around. That is the unique promise, and the importance, of early detection of SMI.

## The Three Faces of Ischemia

Before we get to what you should do next, I want to explore just a little further the link between the risk factors you answered above and SMI. Particularly, if you answered yes to any of the last three questions, pay careful attention!

Most of the medical literature divides the victims of silent ischemia into three, quite distinct, categories: those with no symptoms whatsoever; those who have seemingly recovered from a heart attack in the past; and those with current angina problems. The groups break down approximately like the graph on page 150.

Because each type has separate features and peculiarities, I want to look at them separately.

## No Warning Signs

First are the people with absolutely no symptoms and no history of heart attack (myocardial infarction) or angina.

# AT LEAST 5 MILLION PEOPLE HAVE ISCHEMIA

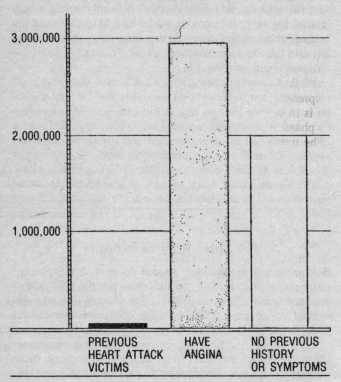

| | PREVIOUS HEART ATTACK VICTIMS | HAVE ANGINA | NO PREVIOUS HISTORY OR SYMPTOMS |

These are the classic cases I described above and certainly the most disturbing ones.

It is hard to know how many such people this includes, but studies from the U.S. Air Force and from Norway estimate it at about 2.5 percent of the population. However, in another study conducted among industrial workers, researchers projected much higher figures: fully 10 percent of the men they studied showed evidence of SMI heart damage.

If these percentages seem abstract, let's bring them down to real life. The lowest possible estimates suggest that some two million Americans are SMI victims—*people who show no heart symptoms whatsoever.* But if the scientists' higher projections are accurate, the true toll may range as high as five to twenty million.

You may wonder, why such a big discrepancy? The real reason is that we do not yet have available any systematic, comprehensive means of knowing how common this phantom is in our general population. But what is clear is that this phantom is far too common for comfort.

The important question, of course, is not one of numbers but of lives—what happens to these people? The Norwegian study I mentioned earlier followed up some two thousand middle-aged men. At first, they found that 2.5 percent of them had undiagnosed, silent ischemic disease. But of more concern was what happened as the years went by. By eight and a half years after the initial study, fully 42 percent of these men had experienced some major cardiac problems—heart attacks, bypass procedures, crippling angina, and the like. If that study applies to our country, the conclusion is indeed serious: More than four out of ten silent ischemic victims are headed straight down the road to major cardiac disaster.

## After a Heart Attack: Still at Risk

The second category on the list includes quite a different group of people. They have had a previous heart attack, but seem to be fully recovered. They show no symptoms of current heart problems, either with angina or other signs. For them, their heart problems would seem to be a chapter in their past.

Unfortunately, we are now learning, that isn't always the case. Many of them continue to suffer silent ischemic damage. Experts estimate that of the approximately 400,000 people who survive heart attacks each year, more than 50,000 of them go on to be haunted by the phantom

## ISCHEMIA AND HEART ATTACKS

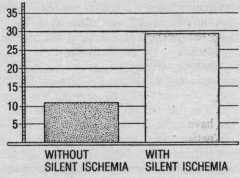

PERCENTAGE OF MORTALITY ONE YEAR AFTER HEART ATTACK

WITHOUT SILENT ISCHEMIA

WITH SILENT ISCHEMIA

of silent ischemia. Put another way, one out of eight heart attack victims will continue to sustain ongoing damage to their heart after a heart attack.

For those who do, the news can be very grim indeed. Having SMI after a heart attack means that you are three times more likely to die, according to a research team from Johns Hopkins Medical Institutions. These scientists examined more than a hundred people who had apparently recovered completely from previous heart attacks. It turned out that 29 percent of the people were suffering silent ischemic attacks. A year later, almost a third of the ones with ischemia were dead of heart failure.

The third and final group of people this phantom haunts is certainly the least surprising. They are the people who already suffer the recurrent chest pain of angina pectoris. Experts estimate that three million Americans fall into this category.

There is one real surprise here, however. It turns out that the angina people can feel is often just the tip of the iceberg. In a recent report in the *American Journal of Medicine*, researchers looked at people suffering from "effort angina"—that is, chest pain during strenuous activity. They found that for every one episode of angina pain these patients know about, they may suffer as many as four silent attacks that they never even notice.

Scientists estimate that 80 percent of people with angina also suffer from frequent episodes of SMI, above and beyond the attacks they recognize. In every one of those silent attacks, the phantom is at work, doing tremendous and hidden harm.

## Diabetics, Beware!

You have seen the three main groups that phantom ischemia patients fall into. But there remains one very important group at risk for this disease, and medical science has only recently begun to understand the link between these people and silent heart disease. The people I am talking about, of course, are those suffering from the insulin disorder diabetes.

Why is it so important? Because the diabetes–heart disease link is quite clear. Over half of diabetics die of heart disease, disease that is often quite advanced before it is discovered. Clearly, it is the phantom of SMI that does this damage, usually without the patients even being aware there is anything wrong with their heart.

Interestingly, this fact supports something many doctors have noticed for some time. Diabetics who come into the emergency room with heart attacks seem much less prone to the strong chest pain that usually accompanies these emergencies. A study from Harvard Medical School reports that diabetics are about three times less likely to suffer pain in heart attacks than the rest of us.

Physiologists have not yet fully explained why this should be so, but it ought to send off a warning flare for you if you have been diagnosed with diabetes. Because if those pain-sensing mechanisms don't work for a full-scale heart attack, they won't work for occasional ischemic episodes, either—and voilà!—the stage is set for this phantom disease to strike.

The moral of this story is an easy one. If you are a

diabetic, it is especially important to bring up the question of silent ischemic heart disease with your doctor.

## Are You a "Have" or a "Have-Not"?

There is no doubt that the tale of this phantom has its dark side—you've already seen that. But, like any good tale, this one also comes with a happy ending, thanks to new research developments.

Your first step is to see whether you are a "have"—that is, you do have some of the risk factors for SMI—or a "have-not." Happily, you can rest comfortably assured that the at-risk groups for SMI are rather well defined. That means that:

- If you don't fit into any of the groups we have talked about
- If you answered no to all the questions in the SMI Risk Profile earlier in this chapter
- If you are generally in good health . . .

. . . then congratulations! If I were you, I would breathe a sigh of relief and skip to the next chapter. You really aren't at very high risk for SMI.

If on the other hand:

- You do see yourself in any of what we've discussed
- You answered yes to any of the Risk Profile questions . . .

. . . then read on. The information in the next few pages may be vital to your health, even your life.

## If I Fit, What Next?

That's easy. Get yourself to your doctor. You can do it the next time you see your own doctor for a routine physical exam. Or, if you are a man over thirty-five years old or a woman over forty-five years old, I would suggest you go pick up the phone right now and make an appointment.

But wait just a second, here. What, after all, is the point of going to a doctor for a condition that comes in episodes, probably won't even occur during the visit, and has no evident symptoms anyway? Good question! (I certainly hope you *did* ask—it shows you've been paying attention!)

What your doctor can do is to order a relatively straightforward test called *ambulatory cardiac monitoring,* or *Holter monitoring,* for short. As you guessed, it isn't always enough to wire you up to a standard electrocardiograph. While that technology can detect the specific electric impulses that signal an SMI attack, research shows that fully half the people with SMI have a normal resting ECG. Even a standard treadmill-type test can also miss this phantom, which, after all, is not usually brought on by exercise. What you really need is a doctor by your side twenty-four hours as you go about your daily life if you are to be assured of the most complete, accurate picture of your heart's activity. Hardly practical, for you or your physician.

Enter the Holter monitor. A small box the size of a Walkman, it fits on a strap around your neck and waist. (That's why some of my patients mistakenly term it a "halter" monitor, instead of Holter, after the scientist who developed it.) This small device packs enough sophisticated electronics to provide a continuous, twenty-four-hour tracking of every beat of your heart. I believe it is the single most common, and most effective, means to isolate and diagnose SMI attacks as they happen.

You can get Holter monitoring from most cardiologists and some clinic- and hospital-based centers. Your own personal family doctor is the first stop to help you find one. It is not inexpensive, and you may spend about two hundred dollars for it. If that seems like a lot of money, believe me, it will be a lot more expensive, in money, anguish, and inconvenience, if you are an SMI victim and don't find out early. Besides, given the new trend toward preadmission testing, since this is done, by definition, outside a hospital, your insurance company may be more than glad to help pay for it.

In some institutions with highly sophisticated radiological departments, you may also be able to find a kind of testing known as *positron-emission tomography*. Although less common, this is another very good way to detect SMI.

But whichever method your physician recommends, the good news to remember about SMI is that if it's there, we now know how to find it. In so doing, you can outfox this phantom at its own stealthy game.

Recognizing this, the American Heart Association has just this month released a recommendation that healthy adults get regular physical check-ups every five years, starting at age twenty. The idea is to start looking specifically for the early warning signs of SMI—before it is too late. That recommendation should remind us all of one crucial fact: The key to defeating this phantom is to steal from it the element of surprise.

## The Easy Part: Treatment

If your cardiologist sees the telltale disturbances in your heart tracing that characterize SMI, you will probably be prescribed one of several kinds of heart drugs. These include the so-called beta-blockers, calcium-channel blockers, or nitrates (including nitroglycerine). Your physician will prescribe one or a combination that helps stabilize the heart rhythm and pumping action.

That, of course, brings us to the happy ending: These drugs usually work, and work well.

## A Note on Nutrition

But this story is not quite over yet. I wouldn't be doing my job if I didn't remind you about the profound dietary factors involved in SMI. This disease, after all, recall, is caused by the same factors that cause most coronary cardiac disease—excess fatty deposits on your artery walls obstructing blood flow. It is all well and fine to take a medicine to help your heart, but how much better, by far, to change how you eat and thus make the drugs unnecessary in the first place.

If you are one of the 60 percent of the SMI patients with a heart history—either angina or heart attack—I hope your doctor has already gone over all of this with you. But if you are in the other 40 percent—the people without any heart disease symptoms at all—you may still need to improve your dietary habits.

By now, the principles of a heart-healthy diet should be well known to everybody, unless you have lived on a desert island for the past ten years (and if you have, you probably don't have to worry, because you've been eating closer to the way Nature intended you to!).

Obviously, we do not have space here to go into the full detail this topic deserves. I really could write a whole book on it (in fact, I did: It's called *How to Be Your Own Nutritionist*). These principles are so important—and so simple—that I will take just a moment to stress the seven major points of a heart-smart diet:

1. Increase your intake of complex carbohydrates or starches (unless you have a yeast infection)
2. Greatly reduce red meats and all animal fats in your diet
3. Increase the amount of fish you eat—try for twice a week
4. When you do eat fats, make sure they are monounsaturated, not saturated or polyunsaturated ones
5. Increase your fiber intake—whole grains, fresh fruits, and vegetables
6. Reduce your intake of highly refined foods
7. Try to avoid refined sugar entirely

Sound familiar? Of course. You will find those same dietary recommendations available from the American Heart Association, the American Academy of Sciences, the Mayo Clinic, Harvard University, the National Cancer Institute—in fact, from every responsible contemporary source of nutritional information.

## A Little Menu-Planning Help

Because we can all benefit from eating heart-smart— whether or not we are a candidate for SMI—I have included a little extra help for making those changes in your eating habits (if you haven't already, that is—or, if you have, and just need a little dietary inspiration). At the end of this chapter you'll find several sample "heart-smart" menus, as well as a list of healthful, helpful heart foods and a list of damaging food items.

Remember, at the beginning of this chapter, how fierce and terrifying this phantom seemed? Well, now that we've come this far, I hope you'll see that this tiger can be tamed. You see, there is really nothing but good news about this phantom. Remember:

• If you are at risk, you will know it.
• If you have it, your doctor can find it.
• If you are diagnosed, you can control it.

Best of all, if you don't have it, you can take real, effective steps to prevent it. I wish that all of our phantoms were so easy!

## Tips for Heart-Smart Eating

Below are the sample menus, good foods and bad foods, for a heart-smart life-style. If you want to know more in detail, you'll find more extensive information in my *How to Be Your Own Nutritionist.* But until then, I hope you'll find these helpful.

## Healthy Heart Menu

**Day One:**

*Breakfast:*
   Low-sodium tomato or vegetable juice
   Oatmeal with cinnamon and apple
   Skim or low-fat milk

*Lunch:*
   Tuna, vegetable salad on whole wheat toast
   Lettuce and tomato
   Pear

*Dinner:*
   Broiled chicken
   Baked potato with yogurt and chives
   Salad of spinach, onions, carrots, mushrooms
   String beans almondine
   Kiwi fruit and berries
   Low-fat, low-sodium cheese

**Day Two:**

*Breakfast:*
   Low-sodium tomato juice
   Whole wheat toast
   Unsweetened jam
   Low-fat yogurt with berries

*Lunch:*
   Vegetarian chili topped with low-fat yogurt
   Tossed green salad
   Banana

*Dinner:*
    Poached salmon
    Brown rice and herbs
    Salad of romaine lettuce, green peppers, tomato,
        alfalfa sprouts or broccoli in garlic sauce
    Pineapple spears and strawberries

## Day Three:

*Breakfast:*
    Carrot juice
    Whole wheat cereal with skim milk
    Blueberries

*Lunch:*
    Carrot and celery sticks
    Sardines in tomato sauce
    Whole-grain crackers
    Peach
    Skim or low-fat milk

*Dinner:*
    Lean veal chops
    Barley pilaf
    Chicory and chopped celery salad
    Steamed baby carrots
    Broiled grapefruit

## Day Four:

*Breakfast:*
    Low-fat cottage cheese
    Grapefruit slices
    Whole wheat bagel

*Lunch:*
    Hearty minestrone soup
    Whole-grain roll
    Skim or low-fat milk
    Plums

*Dinner:*
   Pasta Primavera
   Salad of tomato, cucumber, red onion
   Poached pear

## Day Five:

*Breakfast:*
   Orange juice
   Oat bran with banana
   Skim milk

*Lunch:*
   Low-fat cottage cheese with vegetables and kidney
      beans
   Rice cakes
   Nectarine

*Dinner:*
   Vegetable sticks
   Broiled brook trout
   Parsleyed wild rice
   Fresh spinach and garlic
   Fresh fruit sorbet

## For Dressings Use:

   Vegetable oils
   Low-fat yogurt
   Low-fat cottage cheese
   Vinegar
   Lemon juice
   Garlic
   Onion
   Herbs

## Heart-Smart Foods

| Heart Healers | Heart Breakers |
|---|---|
| Fish high in essential fatty acids:<br>  Salmon<br>  Mackerel<br>  Tuna<br>  Trout<br>  Haddock<br>  Cod<br>Other Fish:<br>  Sole, snapper | Deep-fried fish<br>Fish in cream or butter sauce |
| White meat poultry without skin<br>Lean meats; veal, lean beef | Dark-meat poultry<br>Fried chicken<br>Fatty meats:<br>  Ham, pork, fillet, luncheon meats, hot dogs, bacon |
| Low-fat or skim dairy products<br>Skim milk<br>Low-fat milk<br>Low-fat yogurt and cottage cheese<br>Low-fat low-sodium cheeses | High-fat dairy products:<br>  Cream, regular milk<br>  Half-and-half<br>  Nondairy creamers<br>  Regular fat yogurt<br>  Regular cottage cheese<br>  Regular cheeses<br>  Ice cream |
| Leafy green vegetables<br>Fresh vegetables<br>Fresh fruits<br>Whole grains<br>Beans:<br>  Pinto<br>  Navy<br>  Kidney | Canned vegetables<br>Coconut<br><br>Processed grains<br>Pork and beans |
| Polyunsaturated oils:<br>  Safflower, sunflower, corn | Saturated fats<br>Animal fats<br>Hydrogenated fats<br>Coconut oil, palm oil |

## Heart-Smart Foods

| Heart Healers | Heart Breakers |
|---|---|
| Monosaturated oils: | Salts, soy sauce |
|   Peanut | Mayonnaise, pickled foods |
|   Olive | |
| | Fatty snack foods: |
| |   Chips, candy, cake, |
| |     pastry |

# 9

# Hidden Hypertension:
# Now You See It, Now You Don't

In many respects, this next phantom has a lot in common with the last one. Like SMI, it affects the cardiovascular system, and like that disease, it is part of a major public health problem, affecting tens of millions of Americans. Most of its victims do not know they are at risk. It, too, has the potential to be deadly, but with proper diagnosis and follow-up care, this potential killer is largely controllable. Finally, like the phantom of the last chapter, the key to controlling it involves you, in concert and cooperation with your own physician. But in this case, the phantom is a kind of hypertension—in common English, high blood pressure.

At first glance, it seems hard to imagine what could possibly be "phantom" about this disease. It's hardly as though hypertension were esoteric or unknown. In fact, these days it seems you can hardly turn around without hearing or reading something about it. High blood pressure has been covered thoroughly by everybody from *Newsweek* to the American Heart Association; free blood pressure screenings are available on the street, in the workplace, and at local clinics and hospitals; new discoveries are hailed on the evening news. Thanks to the ballyhoo, there is certainly no doubt that your doctor is well aware of it.

All that is as it should be, because hypertension is among the most common, serious, and treatable of modern-day medical killers. Authorities estimate that about sixty-five million Americans suffer from chronic hypertension, putting them at greater risk for strokes, heart disease, and kidney problems. It has been estimated that high blood pressure directly causes or contributes to a staggering 15 percent of all deaths. So why do I term such a widespread and well-known problem a phantom? The plain answer is that hypertensive conditions are not as simple as they may at first seem. To begin with, there are several different types of hypertension. Most of them remain chronic and relatively stable—you usually either exhibit excessive blood pressure or you don't. The diagnosis is relatively straightforward, not much more complex than taking appropriate measurements with a blood pressure cuff (technically, a sphygmomanometer).

But one variety of hypertension is much less clear-cut. It is called *labile,* or *borderline,* hypertension. (In this chapter, I use the simpler abbreviation, *BHT.*) Both terms mean the same thing: For some reason, your blood pressure does not place you in an immediately evident high-risk group, but it isn't normal either. It may be that you hover right on the border, having a condition that may be on the way to turning into serious, life-threatening hypertension. Or it may be that your blood pressure, instead of remaining relatively stable within a given range, is labile, or changeable, going up and down.

## Hide-and-Seek, But No Game

As I often explain to my patients, it is this "hide-and-seek hypertension" that I classify as the true phantom. But don't let my friendly label fool you—there is nothing remotely amusing about this variety of hide-and-seek. If you have labile hypertension, your blood pressure can sometimes clearly register as elevated, sometimes appear within normal range, sometimes hover between the two, all with little discernible or predictable pattern.

Your blood pressure might happen to be fine at the moment you sit in the doctor's office, the cuff wrapped around your arm. Yet days or even hours later it might be elevated to dangerous levels. The result? You get a "clean bill of health" when in fact you are hiding a disease that puts you at significant risk for the life-threatening complications that come with established hypertension. That is the key—it is not that the borderline hypertension itself poses a particular immediate hazard, but it puts you at much greater risk for going on to acquire sustained, chronic—and very dangerous—hypertension. Scientists estimate that approximately three patients out of ten with the profile of borderline hypertension will go on to manifest classic, established hypertension. Or, to put it in the statistical terms of modern medicine, if you have BHT, your risk for getting chronic hypertension can be as much as three times greater than normal.

This penchant for hide-and-seek is what makes BHT such a deadly phantom adversary and so hard to pin down. The more research physicians do, the clearer it becomes that BHT is a problem distinct from established high blood pressure. The World Health Organization has estimated that as many as one in five adults experience periods of seriously, pathologically elevated blood pressure at some time in their lives (see opposite).

Tragically, almost a third of these victims are in danger of being overlooked longer than necessary—indeed, perhaps never diagnosed—because the telltale signs of their hypertension come and go, falling between the cracks. Now you see why I call it a phantom.

## What Does It Do?

I do not want to suggest that, by itself, BHT poses any particularly exotic risks. In truth, the risks are just the same as with any kind of hypertension—and that makes them plenty serious enough.

Blood pressure is simply the pressure of blood flowing through your veins, arteries, and organs. You can think of

# Approximately 100 Million People Have Hypertension

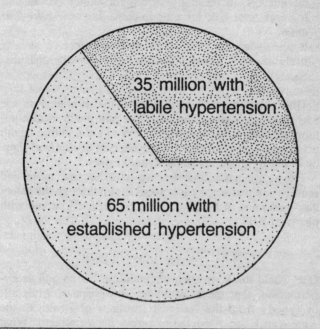

35 million with labile hypertension

65 million with established hypertension

your circulatory system as essentially a highly complex plumbing loop. Like any piping system, it is designed to work at certain pressures. Increase the pressure too much, and the system starts to break down.

In your body, of course, it isn't usually a matter of blowing gaskets or bursting pipes (although this can happen, but that's another story). Instead, when the blood flowing through your arteries is compressed at too high a pressure, you become vulnerable to a laundry list of serious medical emergencies:

- Your heart strains, forced to work harder to pump blood.
- It encourages scarring and growth of fatty deposits in arteries, including vital heart arteries.
- It damages the delicate blood-filtering mechanisms of the kidneys, increasing your risk for kidney failure.
- It raises your risk for a brain-damaging stroke *by four times*.
- It raises your risk for heart failure by *six times*.
- It significantly raises your risk for serious cardiac disease.

  Given such a litany of real problems, it is easy to see why epidemiologists, cardiologists, and public health authorities have targeted hypertension as a top public-health priority. Conscientiously, they have cast a wide and thorough net to locate and treat hypertensives.

  But as we have done so, we have become more and more aware that some cases seem to slip through the safety net—and most of those are the "borderline" people with phantom BHT.

## What Makes It So Slippery?

One would think, in such a "mainline" condition as hypertension, that there would be little dispute. After all, everybody from the National Institutes of Health to the American Heart Association agrees it's a problem. What they can't agree on—as amazing as this may sound—is one general medical definition or precise textbook guideline of exactly what levels constitute true high blood pressure. In part, that is because blood pressure rises steeply with age, so what might be an alarmingly high value for a twenty-five-year-old athlete is well within normal range for her elderly aunt.

  In spite of intensive research on its causes, effects, and patterns, practicing doctors still vary widely in how they define hypertension and even how often they believe patients should be screened for it. To paraphrase the famous

Supreme Court justice, when it comes to hypertension, most doctors "know it when they see it." This gray area is yet another reason the borderline phantom persists.

## The Biology of Blood Pressure

To understand what makes BHT such a phantom, it helps to understand a little about the usual way blood pressure changes, under normal conditions. It is a fact that your blood pressure is constantly in flux, a very adaptive mechanism, from a biological point of view.

Your blood pressure waxes and wanes throughout the day and night, depending on the phase of your body's sleep-awake rhythms (called diurnal cycles) and on factors such as your states of arousal, anxiety, stress, and fatigue; your hormonal levels; even what you had for lunch! Over the course of a day, the "perfect" blood pressure of 120/80 can range by as much as fifty points in the normal run of things. But then usually, like water after a storm, it seeks its own constant level—and this steady state is what you think of as your regular, or *baseline*, blood pressure.

There is also research that suggests that your personality may affect your blood pressure. A Swedish researcher found that patients with BHT tend to be those who suppress their emotions when they feel angry, irritated, or hostile. It's not that they don't feel those things—if anything, the study found, they register these emotions more acutely than others, but they bottle them up. It is a classic cause-and-effect question, and we don't yet know which comes first—the high blood pressure or this emotional style.

In all of this, what should be clear is that your blood pressure is not a fixed, immutable quantity. Rather, it is in motion, responding to your environment. That is one of the reasons it can be so very hard to pin down.

## The Phantom *Sans* Symptoms

There is one other factor that makes it easy for BHT to hide behind its phantom's cloak: It produces virtually no symptoms whatsoever. It is ironic that such a common killer disease, one with such serious consequences, presents such a benign facade, but it does.

This is true not just of BHT, but of almost all kinds of hypertension. Occasionally, people with *very* high blood pressure will have headaches, but that is usually the extent of the symptoms. (Even in people with established hypertension, the overwhelming majority of their headaches have nothing to do with their blood pressure.) Yet this phantom creeps on its stealthy and insidious march, doing its silent damage to your kidneys, arteries, eyes, and brain. By the time it has continued long enough to create symptoms, it is usually much too late to repair the damage that hypertension has wrought.

## If Symptoms Can't Help, Try Statistics

While symptoms may not be terrifically useful to pinpoint this disease, we do have something that can: statistics. We have a rather reliable profile of what groups of people are at highest risk for all sorts of hypertension, including the borderline variety. For example black Americans are about twice as likely to have high blood pressure as whites, and women about one-half to three-quarters as likely as men.

So, the first do-at-home check I recommend is easy. Here's a widely accepted risk-group list, probably the same list used by your own doctor. Where do you rate?

## Hypertension Risks

- Are you a male?                                                        ___
- Are you over forty?                                                    ___
- Are you black?                                                         ___
- Does your family have a history of hypertension?      ___

- Are you more than 20 percent overweight? ___
- Were you overweight as a child? ___
- Do you salt all the food you eat? ___
- Do you have an alcohol problem? ___
- Are you pregnant? ___
- Do you take oral contraceptives? ___
- Is it your style to suppress anger and hostility? ___

There is some debate about how accurately these risk groups target people with high blood pressure, and clinicians are constantly trying to come up with more accurate, more precise categories. Needless to say, nobody would claim that if you are absent from this list, you are 100 percent safe. Or that if you are on it, you are 100 percent doomed to hypertension. After all, statistics is always a game of numbers, of playing the medical odds.

Still, it does mean that if you identify yourself in two or more of the above risk categories, you are quite possibly in the running for blood pressure problems. That's obviously not great news, but what *is* good news is that you have the chance to do something about it.

Some things you can't change—your race, sex, age, and family history. But others you can. I hope that knowing you fall into a hypertension-risk group will be enough to help you make up your mind to take control of the many things on this list you can change—before you suffer the real physiological damage that hypertension can unleash. In hypertension, as in all medicine, you should think of this list as a preventive medicine tool. It's a way not just of knowing your chances but, more importantly, of improving them.

## Accurate Measurements: The Doctor's Dilemma

At this point, you may well be wondering why it is so important to know about risk groups. After all, blood pressure seems wonderfully easy to check. Quick, safe, painless, and risk-free, it only requires us to go to a doctor's office or clinic, let them put the cuff on our arm, and voilà! twenty seconds later, it's done. Would that all medical tests were so easy.

Unfortunately, the more we learn, the more we understand that the situation is a good deal more complicated than that. In what can only be called an exquisite medical irony, research has shown that a physician's office may be one of the single *worst* places to achieve a stable, accurate blood pressure reading. Researchers have discovered that this is due to a reflex called the alerting reaction. A vestige from the days when we lived in the jungles (although, perhaps, still helpful in parts of New York City today!) this reflex kicks into action when you are anxious or aroused.

For some people, the very fact of being in an exam setting and having a physician measure their blood pressure can actually increase their blood pressure significantly—which, of course, produces higher readings!

In one study, the increase in systolic blood pressure attributed to the doctor's presence was, on average, twenty-five points; in some patients, it went as high as seventy-five points! Another study found that the number of patients with high readings varied by more than 100 percent in one reading to the next—with the same patients.

If that's the case, one of my patients once wanted to know, then why not simply adjust readings downward a small amount, to compensate for the alerting reaction? Wouldn't that give an accurate reading? Besides, if being in a doctor's office *increases* your readings, if anything, it could exaggerate the problem and produce a few false alarms. But it wouldn't be likely to miss a hidden blood-pressure problem completely.

Unfortunately, it's not that easy, for several reasons. First of all, the alerting reaction does not work the same way with all people. In the study just mentioned, it would be impossible for doctors to know if they should adjust the readings downward seventy-five points, twenty-five points, or none at all!

Obviously, then, simply compensating randomly for the difference would obscure a significant number of people with real blood pressure problems. For many people, it would be very dangerous, since researchers estimate that 30 percent of people with a one-time high blood pressure reading in their doctor's office do, in fact, suffer from chronic hypertension.

Second, the change from doctor's office to real world doesn't just go in one direction. One study in the *Journal of the American Medical Association* looked at 112 patients who had normal readings in their doctor's offices. Thirty percent of them were, in fact, found to have significantly high blood pressure when they themselves measured it at home. The clear lesson from this and other research is that reliance on one-time, doctor's-office measurements is simply not an effective enough method for detecting BHT.

## There Is No Place Like Home

If something at this juncture sounds familiar, it ought to. It is the same situation we discussed in the last chapter with silent heart disease. In both cases, the best way to track these phantoms is not by measurements outside it.

That's where you come in. There is now a growing research consensus that the best way to get an accurate reading in cases of suspected BHT is to take a series of blood pressure readings spaced throughout the day while you are at home or at work. One recent paper, citing an expert at the University of Michigan, called for at least twenty blood pressure readings outside the medical setting, as well as three high readings in the office, in order to establish a definite blood pressure profile.

Even the most respected medical figures have come to see the immense value of home testing. In the words of one researcher at Oxford University's prestigious Radcliffe Hospital, "Home recordings represent a significant advance in the assessment of blood pressure. [They] should be more widely used in diagnosis and treatment."

What these researchers are saying is that this is one area where you can not only do as well as your doctor, but you can actually do better. It has now been established that an optimal way of getting a handle on floating, phantom blood pressure is to make the patient part of the measuring team. That accomplishes several things at once. Obviously, it removes the variable of stress. You're comfortable, in familiar surroundings instead of being in a foreign, perhaps threatening, medical environment. You minimize the anxiety of having a physician present, because you are the one doing the measuring. It also brings you in as an active, involved partner—and seeing the concrete results gives you a greater incentive for change.

Technical advances have made several reasonably priced (less than fifty dollars) kits that let you take readings easily at home. Some use the traditional blood pressure cuff and stethoscope, others use electronic sensors that give you a readout. (Needless to say, these devices come with explicit instructions for use.) Either way, the entire procedure is quick, painless, and, when carefully done, reliable.

Careful readings over the course of several days will yield a more accurate, more reliable profile of your real blood pressure risk than any one-time spot-check a physician can do in a few minutes in your annual checkup. In this phantom, your cooperation is an absolutely vital, necessary element—a great way you can help your medical team.

While I'm on the subject of self-measurement, let me mention one caveat. Several patients have come to me, concerned after trying those commercial blood pressure meters found in some shopping centers, pharmacies, and other public places. They usually cost fifty cents or a quarter and claim to provide you with a rough guideline of your blood pressure. Used as one-time spot measurements, they have the same possibility for error as any one-time check in a doctor's office. But at least your physician's instruments are likely to be accurate and calibrated, which is not necessarily true of these commercial units. My advice to patients is that, like the video games often found alongside them, these coin-operated gadgets may be fine for entertainment purposes, but for medicine, they fall far short of the mark.

## Once Measured, What Then?

No matter how well you do these measurements, they are obviously not enough by themselves. You should think of them as useful tools for two primary purposes. The first is obvious: to establish whether you are one of the thirty-six million Americans suffering from BHT, so that you can catch this phantom early, before it does its damage.

Second, if you have *already* been diagnosed as hypertensive by your doctor, home testing lets you monitor the progress of your treatment. By creating a "feedback loop," it keeps you informed of what you would otherwise have no way of knowing. Home pressure testing opens a valuable window on your health status, so that you can shape a health program, in concert with your own physician, that subdues this phantom once and for all.

## Put Yourself on the Treatment Team

If you have been diagnosed, there are usually two phases of treatment. The first involves life-style modifications, including the famous four:

1. Lose extra weight (this would be a prudent move by itself, but it will also lower your risk for cancer and atherosclerosis)
2. Restrict salt in your diet
3. Reduce stress
4. Begin a program of regular aerobic exercise

In short, what these do is, one by one, remove you from the risk groups for hypertension we saw earlier—at least those that you can control.

This is the first phase of hypertension control, and for many people, just making these changes is enough to tame their blood pressure.

The second phase is a pharmacological one. Not all patients require it, but for those with dangerously high or unresponsive blood pressure it is an important component of treatment. Your physician may decide your problem is severe enough to warrant a one-two punch, and so put you on any of several blood pressure medications. These are some of the most widely prescribed and effective agents in our entire pharmacopaeia. Most of them have few noxious side effects, and so are quite widely used.

When I explain this to my patients, I find they often raise the same question. Audrey was one, an exceedingly large, jolly woman whose blood pressure problem, I deduced, was at least partially due to her inordinate fondness for high-calorie confections. "But Dr. Berger," she fairly wailed, "if you have a drug that will take care of it, why do I have to give up everything I love? I mean, is it really important? Couldn't I just . . . well, you know, *fudge?*" (I didn't say, as I suspected, that fudge was a part of Audrey's problem—along with cookies, bonbons, and ice cream.) In various forms, I answer this question several times a week.

I will tell you what I told Audrey. It is a basic tenet of medicine to avoid giving medication whenever possible. Drugs are really just the pharmacological equivalent of putting a finger in a straining dike. They are acceptable in a pinch, but it's far better to eliminate the underlying cause. Drugs have side effects, are troublesome, and require medical attention. Often they create problems elsewhere in the body that must, in turn, be handled with more medications. Overeager drug therapy can unleash a whole cycle of drug cross-reactions, which are simply best avoided altogether.

Blood pressure drugs can also be expensive, a significant factor for many people. A recent report in the *American Journal of Public Health* revealed that *more than one in five* lower- and fixed-income Americans cannot afford a steady supply of the necessary hypertension drugs prescribed by their doctor. By their reliance on drugs, they remain at serious risk. To be sure, it is an absolute scandal that our system lets this be the case. But until the system becomes fairer, more equitable, and more humane, there is little doubt that these people would be better off if they could use diet, exercise, and life-style to control their blood pressure. If you are reading this book, you can probably afford such medications. But that still doesn't take you off the hook for trying to make the appropriate life-style changes.

I also remind my patients that making these changes doesn't just help their blood pressure, it improves their entire health. It lowers risk of heart and artery disease and cancer. More to the point, it improves the quality of your life, giving you more vitality, energy, and fewer bouts of illness. In every way, taking these health-positive steps makes you feel better about yourself and your life.

If these weren't reason enough, my last argument against profligate overmedicating is really a philosophical one. This whole book is based on the idea that you are becoming part of your health care team, dedicated to your own wellness and willing to be involved in it. It is a holistic, integrated approach. Clearly, ceding full responsibility to your doctor to hand you a prescription is just the opposite of that attitude. So for all these reasons, when it comes to drugs, I urge my patients to ''just say no''—at least as a first step. Then, only those who really need them will be put on these medications.

## Put This Phantom Behind You

Clearly, the best news of all that you can get out of this chapter is that your blood pressure is one phantom you need not be concerned about. If you aren't in the risk groups, your doctor finds no need for concern, and home testing gives you a clear bill of health, congratulations!

Should any of these, however, suggest that you do have legitimate grounds for concern, I hope you will remember the simple lesson from these pages.

Whether you choose to change the way you live and eat or work with your doctor to make appropriate use of medications, this is one phantom that can be largely eliminated from your life.

I hope this chapter has answered some questions for you. But now, I have one question for you—what are you waiting for?

# 10

# Hypoglycemia: Fad or Phantom?

Human maladies, like hemlines, have a way of going in and out of fashion. A hundred years ago, for example, if you visited your doctor you might well walk out with one of the diagnoses then in vogue: "consumption," say, or "vapors." A century later, in 1988, those same diseases no longer pack our physicians' waiting rooms; they have, in fact, become anachronisms. Yet even with our sophisticated medical system, other diseases continue to drift in and out of the medical spotlight, and of our public consciousness, concern, and awareness, like last year's fashions.

The phantom I want to discuss in this chapter is one of these "fashionable" diseases: hypoglycemia. I suspect that you have already heard a good deal about this phantom. Indeed, it seemed that a few years ago you could hardly pick up a health magazine without reading about this unrecognized syndrome and its many lurking dangers to your health and well-being. In those days, it seemed, every symptom a person had—from everyday fatigue to the slightest mood shift or headache—was easily included under this diagnostic label.

Unfortunately, the very same public awareness that brought so much attention also brought such misinformation, hyperbole, and inaccuracy. Now, fortunately, the medical spotlight has shifted, the excitement has passed, and the dust has settled a bit. Hypoglycemia is no longer the first word on the lips of every one of my patients, the subject of every lurid headline. The public can now examine this disease with a more dispassionate eye.

The medical profession, too, has learned some new things about hypoglycemia and about how and where to look for it. Today, thanks to the wisdom of time, we can now take a closer look at what this phantom is—and what it is not.

Of course, I do not mean to suggest that hypoglycemia is just a fad or fashion. It is a very real, and troubling, condition. Ask any one of the thousands of people who suffer from it. If I didn't believe that, we would not be discussing it here. I also know that it is one disease that clearly meets every criterion for being classified as a phantom:

**It creates nonspecific, systemic symptoms.**
**Its symptoms are often elusive, not able to be pinned down.**
**Its symptoms are too commonly overlooked.**

My point, though, is that it is important to separate where the true phantom leaves off and the popular misconception begins, to distill fact from fiction, and to get an accurate perspective on this disease. For that is the only way you and your doctor can work together productively to pin down, or rule out, this phantom in your own health profile. To help you do that, what follows is a quick overview of our state-of-the-art understanding of this phantom.

## How's Your Greek?

The word *hypoglycemia* is the kind of six-syllable medicalese word that my patients hear and tell me: "That's Greek to me, doctor." Well, in the case of this word, it really *is* Greek! But just in case your ancient Greek is a tad rusty, let's review: *hypo* means "too little"; *gly* is the Greek root for "sugar"; and the suffix *-emia* means "of the blood." String them together, and you have "too little sugar in the blood." (The disease is the polar opposite of diabetes, which creates too much sugar in the blood.)

On its face, perhaps this doesn't sound all that serious. But when you remember that this sugar is what your body uses to fuel every one of its organs and muscles and that without it, all of your body's cells could "run out of juice," you begin to appreciate just how serious low blood sugar can be. Hypoglycemia is, in short, the biological equivalent of a race car running on empty.

Doctors divide hypoglycemia into two main types. The first are quite rare—cases due to a genetic abnormality, alcoholism, liver disease, certain specific cellular disorders, or a cancerous growth in the cells responsible for keeping the sugar balance in your body. But such hypoglycemia—termed *fasting hypoglycemia*—is not the one you've heard all the fuss about.

The syndrome that has received so much popular attention is of another kind, which doctors call *reactive hypoglycemia*. This is a simple imbalance in your body's "sugar circuitry." The name *reactive* means that it occurs in reaction to an event—in this case eating. By definition, its symptoms occur two to five hours after a meal.

The reaction can be due to any of several reasons: Your body cannot properly absorb and assimilate nutrients, your diet is too high in refined carbohydrates, you have had surgery on the gastrointestinal tract, or you have an overactive response of the part of the nervous system controlling your body's reaction to food.

But whatever the cause of this sugar imbalance, the result is anything but sweet. First, the level of sugar in your blood starts to skyrocket. Sensing that rise, your pancreas, the body's sugar thermostat, sounds the alarm, telling its insulin-producing cells to go to work, spilling this hormone into your blood. The insulin will help mop up the excess blood sugar and instruct your liver to act as a great big sugar sponge, soaking up the sugar from your blood and storing it away. But as your body does its best to bring those levels back within bounds, you suffer. When this biochemical brouhaha subsides, your blood sugar levels have plummeted lower than you started with—in fact, below the level your body needs—and you feel the sugar blues, those characteristic symptoms of a hypoglycemia attack.

## Hundreds, Thousands, Millions?

It has become clear over the last few years that we really have little very accurate knowledge of just how many people suffer from true hypoglycemia. Part of the reason for this is that recent studies have shown that the blood tests we have traditionally used—and that were the basis of so many inflated statistics in the popular press over these last few years—have turned out to be less accurate than we once thought.

The standard that has been used for years is the Oral Glucose Tolerance Test, in which a patient drinks a standardized dose of sugar and the doctor scrupulously records blood levels of glucose for several hours. If, when the insulin takes effect, the blood sugar drops below a certain threshold, voilà! you have a diagnosis of hypoglycemia.

Unfortunately, that works better in theory than in practice. In real life, the diagnosis is nowhere near so clearcut. Recent research has shed light on several problems with this approach. First of all, under these laboratory challenge conditions, a large proportion of those people tested will show up in the "too-low" blood sugar range—earning themselves a diagnosis of hypoglycemia—yet seem perfectly healthy, suffering no hypoglycemic symptoms.

A study in the *New England Journal of Medicine* showed that fully one-quarter of perfectly healthy, symptom-free people registered as hypoglycemic on such tests. According to one medical textbook, as many as a third or more of normal people show up as hypoglycemics in four-hour glucose tolerance tests. Such findings have led physicians to wonder whether the glucose tolerance test reveals hypoglycemia or triggers it!

The view from the other side is no more encouraging. A recent Mayo Clinic study looked at 129 patients who suffered from hypoglycemiclike symptoms—and two-thirds of them still passed their tolerance tests with flying colors. The more that clinicians have tested, the more they find that some people can show values lower than the standard hypoglycemia cutoff point yet feel just fine, whereas others score well above the cutoff point and show symptoms. So much for our definitions!

The real lesson here is that we don't have a very good idea of what constitutes an entirely normal level or what blood sugar level defines true hypoglycemia, and that it seems to vary much more than we originally understood. With numbers like this, you begin to understand how easy it is to see this phantom condition when it isn't there.

The bottom line, I believe, is that there are more cases of this syndrome than traditional medicine probably recognizes, and fewer than the astounding numbers claimed by some alternative practitioners. Or, to put it another way, traditional doctors need to learn not to miss hypoglycemia when it is smack under their noses, and alternative doctors, not to see it hiding under every bed. Until then, it will remain underrecognized by one group, overdiagnosed by another, and confusing you, the patient who is stuck in the middle.

## The Hypoglycemic Who's Who

Happily, there is a road out of this confusion. For while there is much we don't know about the "what" of hypoglycemia, there is a lot we do know about the "who"—who is at risk, who gets it, who reports it. I suggest you take a moment to score yourself on this profile:

- Do you have a diabetic in your immediate family?
- Are you more than 20 percent overweight?
- Have you had surgery on your digestive tract or stomach, including a gastrectomy, gastrojejunostomy, pyloroplasty, or vagotomy?

- Have you had a high fever recently?
- Have you been using any antidiabetic drugs, such as insulin?
- Have you gotten unusually intense, strenuous, or pro-longed exercise recently?
- Do you work in a high-stress job or profession?
- Do you drink a significant amount of alcohol?
- Do you consume a significant amount of caffeine (in colas, coffee, or tea) or nicotine, in cigarettes?
- Are you aware of having allergies to certain foods?
- Are you pregnant?

If you find yourself giving several yes answers to the above, you may be in a risk group for developing hypo-glycemia. Of course, these categories are not 100 percent airtight—people having many of these risk factors can be entirely free of low-blood-sugar problems. But each has been linked, in one way or another, with hypoglycemia. And if several of them occur together, it is a good indi-cator that you are at significant elevated risk for the kind of sugar-metabolism problems of hypoglycemia.

There is another side to this "who's who" of hypogly-cemia. The medical literature has reported that the disease disproportionately afflicts younger, white, middle-class fe-males (or people of both sexes) who are young, profes-sional strivers.

As you will see elsewhere in this book, this is a profile that shows up in other phantom diseases as well. But I would just caution you not to take this overly seriously. What it is most likely to reflect is not a biological truth about sugar metabolism but a socioeconomic fact about the people who are most informed about and interested in diseases, who pay close attention to their health, and who have the means to take their complaints to a doctor.

Given the immense media publicity around the hypo-glycemia phantom in the last few years, it is no surprise that the disease is recognized by those people most in touch with that media—and that they are the ones we hear the most about. Particularly in a disease such as this, where the symptoms are rarely debilitating but usually vague and elusive, it is the well-informed, highly motivated patient whose symptoms get recognized. Remember: just because Yuppies may be the tip of the iceberg that comes to physicians' attention, that hardly proves they are the only ones suffering from the problem! If the people in my own practice are any indication, I would say that hypoglycemia affects far more than just this select "risk group."

## Low-Sugar Symptoms

So far we've talked about the mechanism of hypoglycemia and who the people are who are most at risk. But what will be the most helpful for you—what will help you know if this phantom is playing a role in *your* life—is to look at what it does.

As I have said, the symptoms of hypoglycemia are diffuse and nondifferentiated. Many of them could be caused by any number of things—from an ordinary flu, to the vicissitudes of growing older, to a bad day at work—without there being anything at all wrong with your blood sugar.

Among the symptoms most commonly reported as linked to hypoglycemia are the following:

- Chronic intense fatigue
- Muscular tremors, weakness, or shakiness
- Excessive sweating
- Mood swings
- Feeling anxious or keyed up
- Intense hunger
- Recurring headaches (especially at a consistent time)
- Mental dullness and confusion
- Poor concentration, forgetfulness
- Dizziness
- Blurry vision
- Pounding heart or palpitations
- Low sex drive (libido)

## SYMPTOMS LINKED TO HYPOGLYCEMIA

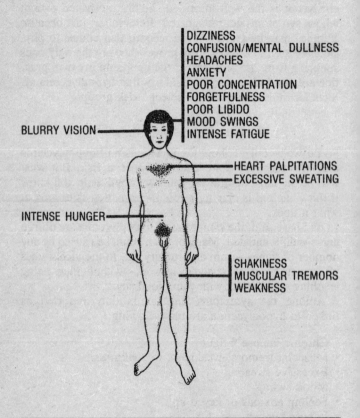

DIZZINESS
CONFUSION/MENTAL DULLNESS
HEADACHES
ANXIETY
POOR CONCENTRATION
FORGETFULNESS
POOR LIBIDO
MOOD SWINGS
INTENSE FATIGUE

BLURRY VISION

HEART PALPITATIONS
EXCESSIVE SWEATING

INTENSE HUNGER

SHAKINESS
MUSCULAR TREMORS
WEAKNESS

But in addition to these more common and immediate symptoms, there is some evidence that hypoglycemia can also be an exacerbating factor in a range of other, more serious diseases. One medical almanac article states that the low-blood-sugar syndrome can contribute to illnesses as varied as epilepsy, ulcers, asthma, impotence, allergies, and arthritis. In addition, the psychological effects of low blood sugar can mimic, or aggravate, such symptoms of mental illness as depression, learning disorders, and insomnia.

A research paper published in the British medical journal *The Lancet* found an even more serious side effect of hypoglycemia. The doctors studied 794 pregnant women and found that hypoglycemia was significantly associated with reduced growth of the fetus, complications of pregnancy, and even directly related to untimely fetal death.

## Three Steps to Diagnosis

By now it should be obvious: The health consequences of this phantom can be quite profound. Hypoglycemia can affect your energy, your mental abilities, your work productivity, your sex life, your heart, your mental health, even the well-being of your fetus. For all these reasons, it is a problem that requires accurate and timely diagnosis.

Yet as we have seen, that is more easily said than done. First of all, many medical practitioners still do not take this malady seriously enough. I remember how one of my patients, Dierdre, put it, "When I asked my doctor about it, I got the feeling he doesn't see much of a difference between hypoglycemia and hypochondria!" What Dierdre put her finger on is, unfortunately, all too true. Far too many practitioners still relegate this syndrome to the waste can of "neurosis" and "malingering" instead of recognizing it for the demonstrable, biochemical illness it is. (It's strange, when you think about it. No doctor could pass his or her medical boards if he or she didn't take seriously the disease of diabetes, which is, after all, simply the reverse side of the blood sugar coin. That disease is universally recognized as a serious and very real problem, even a lethal one. Yet for some reason, its blood sugar brother, hypoglycemia, has yet to be taken as seriously by the medical community.)

But even assuming that your own doctor is well informed and interested and is looking for hypoglycemia in good faith, the standard means of diagnosing it—the five-hour glucose tolerance test—is very flawed, as we have seen.

So how can you be sure of really tracking down this phantom if it is there, playing a role in your own health? There are three main ways, two of which require your doctor's help and one that doesn't. All rely on the most recent medical thinking, which is focused on a more natural, real-life approach to measuring blood sugar, instead of an artificial, laboratory-induced approach.

Since we have seen that there is so much variability in the results of the glucose tolerance test, some authorities now think it is better to replace it with another kind of blood measurement. This involves not a staggered series of blood samples but only one, drawn after a balanced, normal meal.

This new method relies on a simple idea: If the artificial conditions of the glucose tolerance tests—involving fasting, then a massive dose of sugar—can actually *create* hypoglycemic results in normal people, what we need to measure instead is what happens under the normal nutritional conditions of your own body. The simplest way is simply to do what Nature intended you to: eat a standard, balanced meal and then watch what your body does by itself. If, under those circumstances, you register very low on blood sugar, it is a fair bet that that is an accurate reflection of what is happening to you after every meal.

The second way to test also involves only one measurement, but it is somewhat trickier. It involves getting a blood test at a time *when you are actually experiencing symptoms*. Again, the idea is to get a representative slice of real life, not to create an artificial laboratory situation. If your blood sugar profile is perfectly normal yet you are having noticeable symptoms, it tells you and your doctor to look elsewhere for their cause.

## The Nosh Test

The third means of testing doesn't require your doctor's help at all. You can do it all on your own—with a little help from your kitchen. Remember that the symptoms of low blood sugar come as a response to the insulin that is released after you eat food. So it follows that you can use this link as a test.

The next time you experience what you think might be hypoglycemia-related symptoms, try this pleasant experiment: Eat a little something. (What we New Yorkers call a nosh.) The best thing would be a low-sugar, high-protein item, such as a handful of nuts or some low-fat, unsweetened yogurt. If, after eating, you feel your symptoms subside, it suggests that your problems may indeed be due to an oversensitive food-insulin-blood-sugar thermostat.

One note of caution, though. Don't make your snack something heavy in refined sugar or simple carbohydrates (ahem—put that Twinkie back in the wrapper!). Because these food items release their sugar so quickly, they will just start you off on another boom-bust sugar cycle. What you want is a time-release food such as protein or complex carbohydrates, which will not only gradually pull you out of your sugar slump but *keep* you out!

## Now for the Easy Part

In banishing the hypoglycemia phantom, as with so many of its phantom cousins, the hardest part is figuring out what ails you. From then on, treating it is easy. Or, in this case, I should say living with it, because the best Rx for this phantom is really one of simple dietary vigilance and awareness.

The principles of blood sugar fitness are really very simple, and they all rely on one basic principle: Eat to smooth out the peaks and valleys of the sugar-insulin-hypoglycemia cycle. To do that, here are the six steps to blood-sugar health that I recommend for all my patients with a low-blood-sugar problem.

*Step One: Adopt a diet higher in protein, lower in carbohydrates, and with only a moderate amount of fat.*

In general, the average American diet breaks down like this:

## The Average American Diet

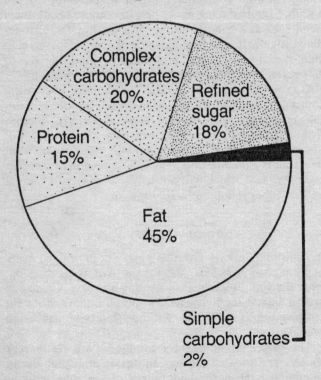

# The Optimal Basic Diet and Hypoglycemic Diet

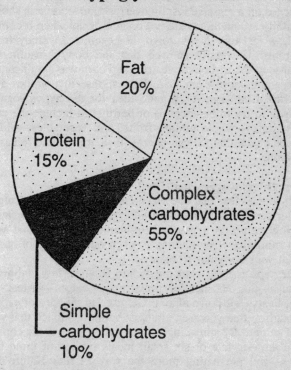

As I wrote in my last book, *How to Be Your Own Nutritionist*, the optimal basic diet for most of us looks very different (see above).

For hypoglycemics, this proportion is particularly important. Keep the protein at 15 percent of your calories, because this is the most time-released of any energy source. Try to keep your level of dietary fat at 20 percent, as well.

*Step Two: Eat slow-absorbing carbohydrates rather than fast-absorbing ones.*

This is another way to slow down the sugar rush that touches off a massive insulin overreaction. Research shows that all carbohydrates are not created equal when it comes to how fast they break down. For example, a study from Stanford University showed that the body's insulin response to the carbohydrates rice and corn was significantly lower and more even than the response to potatoes and gelatin. Likewise, it's a good idea for the hypoglycemic person to try to balance his or her diet to include the carbohydrates—whole grains, fruits, and vegetables—which break down their sugar energy in a more time-released fashion.

*Step Three: Graze, don't stuff.*

It seems clear that one way to take yourself off the sugar roller coaster is to redesign your eating pattern. Because hypoglycemia is a reactive problem, it follows that you can minimize it by helping to even out the load of sugar input your body has to react to.

Try spacing out your meals into smaller, less elaborate snacks—the "noshes" I spoke about before—instead of big, hearty, sit-down affairs. Get used to the idea of eating enough so that you aren't hungry but not so much that you feel stuffed. By spreading your calories out over the course of a day—in five or six small meals instead of three big ones—you are eating more the way Mother Nature intended you to. Your body evolved over millions of years to respond to food in small quantities on a regular basis. Sticking closer to that schedule will lower the strain on your system—and reduce your symptoms.

*Step Four: Wave good-bye to junk food.*

Let's face it—you should have done this anyway. But if you think you have possible hypoglycemic symptoms, it's crucial. Most of the highly refined, sugary foods on the junk food racks pack a wallop of hyperconcentrated sugar.

Believe me, from a biochemical point of view, these "sweet nothings" could challenge the sugar thermostat of an elephant! From the point of view of your pancreatic insulin-producing cells, every bite of these sticky-sweet confections throws them into high-stage, flat-out red alert, in a biochemical panic to combat the infusion of high-power sugars. The wild gyrations of sugar and insulin put a tremendous strain on your pancreas and other organs, sending your energy level through the roof, then bringing you crashing down again—the sugar-rush/sugar-blues syndrome. In short, there is no better way to assure the sugar boom-bust cycle than to eat these things—and no better way to minimize those problems than by avoiding them altogether. Enough said.

*Step Five: Reduce caffeine, alcohol, tobacco.*

This is closely related to the last principle. Since hypoglycemia is a disease of unnecessary ups and downs, you want to minimize the causes of these fluctuations. Getting rid of artificial stimulants is the best way to do this. Many people with low blood sugar have gotten themselves into a dangerous energy-depleting pattern of eating wrong, plummeting into a hypoglycemic attack, then taking stimulants to pick themselves up—just so that they can do it all over again. The casual way in which our culture uses stimulants can easily mask the underlying problems that need your real attention—an improper diet. Worse, the cycle of low blood sugar and high stimulant puts a real strain on several of your most important organs and physiological systems, including adrenal glands, stomach, nervous system, and cardiovascular system. If you can cut these stimulants completely out of your life, you'll be doing yourself a big favor.

If not, there are ways to minimize the damage they can do. Alcohol, for example, is very closely related to hypoglycemic problems—in heavy drinkers, low blood sugar can even be the primary cause of the disease. In a way, that's hardly surprising, because alcohol is a highly concentrated form of calories, sugars, and toxins that your body has to process.

Some people aggravate that damage by consuming their alcohol in combination with very sweet mixers or additives. That rum and Coke or that sticky-sweet daiquiri may taste delicious, but they represent a serious one-two punch for your sugar-balancing system. Try cutting down on them, perhaps switching to a simpler drink, such as wine or beer. And anytime you drink, make sure you are eating a little something at the same time. That food—particularly if it contains protein, such as peanuts or other nuts—helps slightly even out the sugar-absorption curve, and so minimizes your symptoms.

*Step Six: If you are overweight, reduce.*

We know that being overweight—that is, more than 20 percent over your ideal body weight—is related to sugar disorders of all kinds, including diabetes and hypoglycemia. Of course, you should lose that weight for a lot of other reasons. It will help your heart, arteries, and kidneys, not to mention your sex life and social circle! But it may also help lower your risk for the boom-bust sugar cycle of hypoglycemia.

Not all of the medical establishment agrees on the validity of all six of these principles. Some researchers claim that eating lightly, increasing the protein in your diet, and having more frequent meals only serve as placebo effects. They reason that, while their patients may report feeling better, there is no 100 percent demonstrable link.

I don't put much stock in that argument. First of all, if you feel better, it doesn't really matter why. An improvement based on a placebo effect is still an improvement! Besides, the standard of a hypoglycemic diet like the one I describe conforms to everything we know about the physiological processes of the sugar-regulation cycle, and it is widely used in clinical practice.

Finally, these are dietary changes that can't hurt, and if you are one of those people haunted by the low-blood-sugar phantom, they have the potential to turn your life and health completely around! So, for all these reasons, I say try it . . . you might like it.

## To Get You Started . . .

In order to help you get a feel for an optimal hypoglycemic diet, I have included below a sample few days' worth of sugar-smart meals, as well as lists of the best and most appropriate foods to keep your blood sugar level in control.

The suggestions below conform to the principles we have discussed. By using them, you can literally eat your way out of the low-sugar symptoms that may now be plaguing your life. Good luck—and *bon appétit!*

**Food Lists:**

- *Animal protein.* Fish, fowl, or other animal protein is okay, but preferably one with low fat. Stay away from heavily fatted beef and pork cuts, as well as all processed foods.
- *Vegetables* should be eaten as fresh as possible. If not raw, then lightly steamed or stir-fried with little oil.

| | |
|---|---|
| Artichokes | Lettuce |
| Asparagus | Mushrooms |
| Avocados | Okra |
| Bean sprouts | Olives |
| Beets | Onions |
| Broccoli | Parsley |
| Brussels sprouts | Peppers |
| Cabbage | Pimientos |
| Carrots | Pumpkin |
| Cauliflower | Sauerkraut |
| Celery | Spinach |
| Chives | Squash |
| Cucumbers | String beans |
| Eggplants | Tomatoes |

- *Fruits are fine.* Feel free to eat two servings a day. When possible, they are best eaten raw to enjoy their full ripeness and succulence.

| | |
|---|---|
| Boysenberries | Nectarines |
| Cantaloupe | Papayas |
| Cranberries | Peaches |
| Grapefruit | Strawberries |
| Lemons/limes | Tangerines |
| Melons | |

- *Nuts and seeds* must only be eaten raw, unsalted, unsmoked, and unprocessed.
- *Dairy products* can be loaded with fat. Choose skim milk, low-fat yogurt, and low-fat cheeses.
- *Breads* are a good source of necessary whole grains. Avoid highly processed and refined white bread.
- *Beverages* can include juices, water-decaffeinated coffee, plain soda, and mineral water. Fruit juices are highly concentrated sugars—avoid them.

## Hypoglycemic Menus

**Day One:**

*Breakfast:*
   Soft-boiled egg
   Whole wheat toast
   Skim or low-fat milk

*Snack:*
   Whole-grain crackers
   Apple

*Lunch:*
   Chef salad
   Melba toast

*Snack:*
  Carrot sticks
  Low-fat cottage cheese

*Dinner:*
  Tossed green salad
  Broiled chicken
  Brown rice
  Zucchini and tomato

*Snack:*
  Strawberries
  Pecans

**Day Two:**

*Breakfast:*
  Oatmeal
  Blueberries
  Skim or low-fat milk

*Snack:*
  Rice cakes with nut butter
  Banana

*Lunch:*
  Sliced turkey sandwich with lettuce and tomato

*Snack:*
  Cucumber spears
  Low-fat yogurt dip

*Dinner:*
  Endive salad
  Lean steak
  Baked potato
  Steamed broccoli

*Snack:*
   Nectarine
   Popcorn

## Day Three:

*Breakfast:*
   Whole-grain cereal
   Skim or low-fat milk
   Strawberries

*Snack:*
   Almonds
   Pear

*Lunch:*
   Spinach salad
   Whole-grain roll

*Snack:*
   Celery sticks with cashew butter

*Dinner:*
   Spinach salad
   Broiled flounder
   Wild rice
   String beans almondine

*Snack:*
   Tangerine

## Day Four:

*Breakfast:*
   Whole wheat bagel
   Butter
   Unsweetened jam

*Snack:*
   Whole-grain crackers
   Melon

*Lunch:*
   Cottage cheese and fruit platter
   Rice cakes

*Snack:*
   Green and red pepper slices
   Low-fat cheese

*Dinner:*
   Broiled veal chop
   Whole-grain roll
   Peas and carrots
   Spinach and garlic

*Snack:*
   Peach
   Pecans

## Day Five:

*Breakfast:*
   Poached egg
   Whole wheat toast

*Snack:*
   Rice crackers with unsweetened jam

*Lunch:*
   Tuna plate with vegetables
   Whole-grain crackers

*Snack:*
   Raw broccoli and cauliflower
   Low-fat cottage cheese and chives

*Dinner:*
    Tossed green salad
    Pasta and red clam sauce
    Asparagus spears

*Snack:*
    Apple
    Walnuts

# 11

# The Women's Phantom: Premenstrual Syndrome

You may recall that when I first introduced the family of phantom diseases, I said that, as a class, they tend to have a "sexist" streak. By that I meant that they generally prey on women more often than on men. Not all of them are that way, of course. Certain of them, like the cardiovascular phantom of labile hypertension, do show a distinct preference for males.

But this chapter is devoted to a phantom that is the worst sort of sexist, for it always attacks women, and only women. It is the much-discussed, long-familiar, yet ever-elusive phantom of premenstrual syndrome, or PMS.

Given its long history, it is somewhat surprising that we do not know more about PMS than we do. It was more than fifty years ago, in 1931, that researchers first described the wide emotional and psychological disturbances it can create. A few years later, in 1934, another paper was published showing that the syndrome could also unleash a wide range of physical symptoms. So for more than a half century, we have known about PMS. Yet, for all that time, it has managed to remain something of a medical enigma.

That long history was summed up recently, in the words of two researchers writing recently in the journal *American Family Physician:* "Although the medical literature on PMS has grown significantly since the disease was first described, there is still no convincing evidence on the etiology, evaluation, and treatment of the disorder.'' In other words, despite our years of effort and volumes of ink that have been spilled over this perplexing phantom, we remain largely in the dark about what truly causes it and what to do about it. That situation is precisely what makes PMS such a classic phantom disease.

As we explore it on these next pages, I hope you will keep one thing in mind: Although it may be a phantom, that doesn't mean there's nothing you can do about it. If you are one of the many millions of women who suffer from mild to severe PMS symptoms, I want you to know that it is not a lost cause, that you should not resign yourself to ''just learning to live with it.'' I don't accept that, and neither should you. Together, in this chapter, we can take a look at what facts we do know and try to put them to work for you.

## What Is This Phantom?

On the face of it, the definition of PMS is deceptively simple: It includes the physical, emotional, and behavioral changes that occur for women in the few days before their monthly period. That much almost everybody agrees on.

But underneath that simple definition lies a Pandora's Box of medical controversy. There is no better way of illustrating that than to look at the most basic statistic for any disease: its incidence. Or, to put it in plain English, how many people it touches. In a medical textbook, that is always one of the very first, basic pieces of information you find about any disease. It is usually fairly straightforward and clear.

Not so with PMS. Take a look at the confusion, even among the experts:

> The general consensus is that 20–40% of women of childbearing age are afflicted . . . of them, possibly 5 to 10 per cent have such severe PMS that it disrupts families and society (Zaren Chakmakjian, ''A Critical

Assessment of Therapy for the Pre-Menstrual Tension
Syndrome," *Journal of Reproductive Medicine*, Aug.
1983, Vol. 28, No. 8, p. 532).

Pre-menstrual changes have been reported to affect 20
to 60 per cent of the female population (Uriel Halbreich,
"The Clinical Diagnosis and Classification of Premenstrual Changes," *Canadian Journal of Psychiatry*, Nov.
1985, Vol. 30, p. 489).

PMS, to one degree or another, besets an estimated 40
per cent of women during their reproductive years . . .
five to six million women experience symptoms severe
enough to disrupt their personal and work routines
(*Harvard Medical School Health Letter*, Aug. 1984, Vol.
IX, No. 10, p. 1).

PMS . . . affects up to 40 to 60% of women between
the ages of 15 to 50. Some 12 to 15 million women
suffer from this disorder in the United States alone (Har-
riet Greveal, M.D., "Answers for PMS," *Total Health*,
Jul. 1985, p. 26).

Surveys of menstruating women have indicated that between 70 and 95 per cent notice one or more . . . symptoms (Jane Brody, "Treatment Techniques Vary for
Pre-Menstrual Syndrome," *The New York Times*, Apr.
16, 1986, p. C5).

Eighty to ninety per cent of women have at least one
premenstrual symptom, and of that thirty to forty per
cent have symptoms severe enough to disrupt their life-
style (Mary Laughlin, M.D., and Ramona Johnson,
M.D. "Pre-menstrual Syndrome," *American Family
Physician*, Mar. 1984, p. 265).

It has been estimated that 95% of American women suffer from premenstrual symptoms at one time or another.

[Our study shows] thirty nine per cent had premenstrual tension (Hamish Sutherland, "A Critical Analysis of Pre-Menstrual Syndrome," *The Lancet*, June 5, 1965, p. 1180).

These represent only a tiny slice of the professional and popular literature available on PMS, but I think you get the idea.

The more of these journal articles and learned papers I study, the more I am convinced of two basic facts. First, even the authorities don't agree on the scale and scope of this problem. Second, behind the statistical smokescreen, PMS is a very real and potentially a very devastating condition.

Unless you are trained in biostatistics and epidemiology, I doubt that such percentages mean a lot to you. So let's bring them down to more concrete, human terms. The woman between the ages of fifteen and fifty who has not experienced some degree of PMS is a very lucky exception, for almost every other woman has at some point, or does on a regular basis. The problems fall roughly into three general types: behavioral, physical, and emotional.

But whatever the type, they wreak havoc in many millions of women's lives. According to the statistics, severe PMS may affect as many as four women out of ten in this age range—or about twenty-five *million* American women. For them, PMS can be a severe, at times crippling, malady. According to a recent Harvard University publication, five or six million women in our country have such severe PMS symptoms that it disrupts their personal and work routines. PMS can throw its long shadow over every other aspect of their lives, as well—in their career, with their loved ones and families, even in normal social interactions. One recent study found that more than one-quarter of the women surveyed had severe enough symptoms to have sought a doctor's help.

## Murderers and Parakeets

Despite the growing public awareness of PMS, some people still pooh-pooh this disease. They seem to view it as conscious malingering, a condition belonging to neurotics and hypochondriacs. I think that indicates a profound ignorance about the depth of the disturbances PMS can cause. Not that it always does, mind you—by far the majority of women with PMS tolerate its symptoms fairly well.

But for some, it can drive them over a very dangerous brink. This is how a noted British specialist in PMS described the condition in a classic article in the *British Medical Journal* of May 9, 1953: "The premenstrual syndrome may seriously interfere with work and social activities, and can be incapacitating." In that country, there have been three cases where women successfully pleaded they had "diminished responsibility" for violent actions—including one attempted murder—committed in the throes of PMS. While that defense has not stood in American courts, even a quick look at case reports in the PMS literature testifies to what a sad and disrupting influence the condition can be for many women.

One psychiatric review recently reported four severe PMS cases in which women hit their children, argued violently with their spouses, and had hallucinations during PMS episodes. One woman even strangled her five-year-old son's pet parakeet in a fit of impulsive rage!

When I look at the statistics on PMS, when I hear case histories like the ones above, and when I count the numbers of women in my own practice with moderate to severe PMS problems, I cannot call it a fable, a fancy, or a fad. I cannot help but suspect that if this were happening to men, it would be called an epidemic, pure and simple. In my opinion, that's exactly what it is, and that's why PMS deserves to be taken very seriously by our medical establishment.

## The Roots of PMS

At this point, it seems reasonable to inquire as to the underlying causes behind PMS. Unfortunately, any discussion on that subject is likely to be either very long or very short. Long, in the list of possible mechanisms that doctors and researchers have advanced in the last fifty years to account for the broad spectrum of PMS symptoms. Short, in that, when all is said and done, we still have no definitive cause for this phantom.

At various times, doctors have suggested causes ranging from diet (too little Vitamin $B_6$ or magnesium, or too much caffeine) to hormones (too much of the female hormone estrogen, or too little of another hormone, progesterone). Others have laid the cause of PMS to faulty sugar metabolism, problems with the hypothalamus and pituitary glands, imbalances in the brain's neurotransmitters, the immune system, and even psychosocial suggestion.

My own view is that, as we further plumb the mysteries of PMS, we will see that many of these factors may be at work. Most likely, there is a complex, interrelated web, involving neurological, endocrine, and perhaps immunologic influences, each acting on the other systems. But through it all, what is clear is that we have a long way to go before we will truly unravel the complexities of this syndrome.

## How This Phantom Hides

It certainly seems strange that, for a disease that is so widespread and that leaves such a significant imprint on so many lives, the medical machine is not better able to track it down, find its cause, and know when it is there and when not. But we aren't, can't, and don't.

This points to a glaring loophole in our vision of the best way to conduct medicine. Usually, we require that a disease present itself in clearly delineated diagnostic categories. For certain diagnosis, we rely on specific blood, urine, and other biochemical tests. Armed with these results, and only then, are we willing to label diseases. That system works fairly well much of the time, because it corresponds fairly well with the way diseases often occur in the world.

But this isn't always so. In the case of PMS, in fact, it isn't the case at all. This syndrome doesn't present itself all neatly wrapped up with clear and consistent signs and symptoms. It doesn't always come out looking the same way, even in the same person. Most of all, it doesn't oblige us with telltale biochemical changes that we can test, measure, compute.

At present, just as we don't know what causes it, we have no reliable and specific biochemical, physiological, or psychological tests to pick up PMS. So, even if your doctor suspects that that is what may be going on, he or she can't call up a laboratory and order a test that will pin it down in black and white, beyond any shadow of a doubt.

Needless to say, that represents something of an uncomfortable dilemma for doctors hobbled by the confines of our test-based medical model. Some practitioners still subscribe to the old "if-I-can't-test-for-a-problem-it-isn't-there" attitude. To an extent, that is just the reasonable caution of a physician who is taught to distrust what he cannot see. When that attitude helps avoid needless, dangerous treatments, it is a good and useful one. But when it blinds us to what is right in front of us, including our patients' suffering, it does nobody any good.

Today, after so much attention in both the popular and the professional literature, most doctors will agree that *something* is certainly going on here. Few physicians can, in good faith, ignore this syndrome, for it is simply too common, and its effects too widespread. But they may still not know just how to approach it, because it is such a different phenomenon from the diseases they are used to treating.

The result? A syndrome that, like few others, falls

smack between the medical cracks—a classic, no-doubt-about-it phantom, *par excellence*.

## Slippery Symptoms

With most of the phantoms we have seen so far, we have at least been able to pinpoint them through their symptoms. That is less straightforward with PMS, simply because the range of symptoms is so broad. Most authorities report about 150 different symptoms associated with this syndrome. Some cite as many as 200! While I don't want to give the whole laundry list here, I do want to reprint one list given by two scientists from the Biological Psychiatry branch of the National Institute of Mental Health. I believe this list covers the principal symptoms that are likely from PMS. The NIMH researchers break down their list of PMS symptoms into nine distinct categories:

**Mood:**
Sadness
Anxiety
Anger
Irritability
Mood swings

**Pain:**
Headache
Breast tenderness
Joint and muscle pain

**Autonomic nervous system:**
Nausea
Diarrhea
Palpitations
Sweating

**Appearance:**
Acne
Greasy hair
Dry hair

**Mental function:**
Reduced concentration
Indecisiveness
Paranoia
Oversensitivity to rejection
Suicidal thoughts

**Fluids:**
Weight gain
Bloating
Puffiness and edema
Excessive urination

**Central nervous system:**
Clumsiness
Seizures
Dizziness
Numbness
Tremors

**Behavioral:**
Reduced motivation
Poor impulse control
Social isolation
Reduced efficiency

**Other:**
Insomnia
Excessive sleeping
Loss of appetite
Binge craving and eating
Fatigue
Lethargy
Agitation
Changes in sex drive

What I hope is obvious, even from this abridged list, is that there is virtually no area of your life—from your sexual satisfaction to your appearance to your job performance—that this phantom does not have the potential to disrupt.

Happily, no PMS sufferer exhibits this full range of symptoms, certainly not all at the same time. There is a much shorter list of the most common symptoms, according to researchers at the Mayo Clinic and Harvard Medical School.

The primary culprits include the following:

1. Fatigue
2. Depression
3. Headaches
4. Mood swings
5. Crying spells
6. Bloating (especially abdominal)
7. Breast swelling and tenderness
8. Junk food binges
9. Constipation
10. Clumsiness
11. Irritability
12. Anxiety
13. Hostility

There you have it, the "unlucky thirteen" roster of PMS symptoms.

Some of the purely physical symptoms of PMS are illustrated opposite.

Before we leave the subject of symptoms, there is one, less-often discussed side of PMS symptoms you may not know about. All of the popular literature and most of the professional papers tend to stress the negative sides of PMS symptoms, such as the lists of unpleasant effects you saw above. But a small percentage of women also report significant positive changes associated with PMS. For those women, the final days before their menses may bring an exhilarating period of higher energy and efficiency, stronger sex drive, powerful feelings of affection, and heightened attention and concentration. To be sure, such "PMS positives" are more the exception than the rule. But if you are one of the few fortunates who experience these little-talked-about advantages of PMS, you should count yourself tremendously lucky!

## Even the Experts Can't Agree

You might think that a syndrome with so many symptoms would be impossible to miss, but in fact, the reverse is true. Because of the immense variability of the symptoms of PMS in your body, most physicians cannot come to a generally accepted consensus of exactly what symptoms you have to manifest in order to be diagnosed for PMS and treated accordingly. The disagreement is further exacerbated by the fact that none of the symptoms is highly specific to this syndrome and may often be caused by other problems, including ovarian cysts, uterine fibroids, endometriosis, and pelvic inflammatory disease.

Some evidence even suggests that which of the various PMS symptoms you manifest depends in part on underlying factors within your own medical and psychological makeup. For instance, women previously diagnosed with specific psychological problems—such disturbances as depression, antisocial behavior, or paranoia—may find that those symptoms get worse during an episode of PMS.

## PHYSICAL TRACES OF PMS

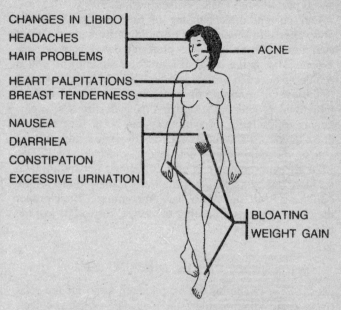

CHANGES IN LIBIDO
HEADACHES
HAIR PROBLEMS

ACNE

HEART PALPITATIONS
BREAST TENDERNESS

NAUSEA
DIARRHEA
CONSTIPATION
EXCESSIVE URINATION

BLOATING
WEIGHT GAIN

## PMS RELATED TO MENSTRUAL PERIOD

PMS WINDOW

FOLLICULAR PHASE    LUTEAL PHASE

Likewise, if you are troubled by acne, or recurrent cold sores (herpes virus infections), they may worsen during the few days immediately preceding your regular menstrual period—the PMS "danger period."

Our current understanding of premenstrual problems now takes into account this extraordinarily wide gamut of symptoms. That's why the preferred label is now *syndrome*. That is the medical term for a situation in which problems occur in groups and bunches. In a syndrome, it is the overall grouping of symptoms that counts, not the individual problems themselves. In such diseases, a particular constellation of symptoms can occur together, but don't have to. (The most infamous of such syndromes, of course, is autoimmune deficiency syndrome, or AIDS. Like all syndromes, it is usually defined not by any one problem but by a group of symptoms.) That, in fact, is the one thing PMS and AIDS have in common: Their proper diagnosis depends on seeing the forest, instead of just the trees.

## Not the "Whats," the "Whens"

Most of the phantoms we have looked at so far are relatively easily diagnosed by the "whats"—what you feel, what your doctor finds on tests. But as we have seen, with PMS, your specific symptoms really don't help very much to define and determine this syndrome.

In order to really track down PMS, you also need to know the "whens." As its name indicates, PMS symptoms are intimately tied to the natural rhythms of your body's menstrual changes. In that respect, PMS has a very specific identifying fingerprint. It always happens during a very specific time, usually the few days or week immediately before your period. This is what biologists term the *luteal phase* of your menstrual cycle, after your body has ovulated but before monthly bleeding occurs—that is, the second two weeks of the menstrual cycle. (The first two weeks, before ovulation, is termed the *follicular phase.*)

In the last days of this phase, just before a woman's monthly bleeding, is the time I call the *PMS window,* when symptoms are most likely and most severe. Classically, PMS symptoms are dramatically reduced or disappear completely with the arrival of your monthly bleeding. Because the syndrome waxes and wanes on such a rigid schedule, this can be your single best clue for determining if what you are suffering from is truly PMS.

One clear indicator of how much PMS symptoms keep to a schedule is reflected in some news that broke just this week as I sat down to write this. The American Psychiatric Association just announced a "new" disorder, now included in their most recent diagnostic manual. The disease is termed *late luteal phase dysphoric disorder.* That is simply a fancy, medicalese name to denote the mood and emotional changes of what we know as PMS. The label underscores what we already know about the "whens" of PMS. It occurs late in the luteal phase, and one of its prime symptoms is dysphoria, from the Greek word meaning "distressed"—in today's psychiatric parlance it means the state of being anxious, depressed, or restless. This fancy three-dollar diagnostic label is just a fancy way of saying what millions of women experience firsthand every month: the telltale signs of PMS.

Knowing the "whens" of PMS is absolutely crucial to determining if you have it. As I tell my patients, making that determination is crucial, for several reasons. Because the free-floating, on-and-off symptoms of PMS can also suggest many other, more serious disorders, it is important to rule out PMS as a possible cause before going on to look for more complex or medically significant possibilities. Also, because many of the symptoms involve your mind, mood, energy, and emotions, it can be very reassuring and reaffirming to know that they do, indeed, have a biological basis in PMS.

I recently saw a woman patient, Wendy V., who started

crying in my office when I told her I suspected PMS. "Dr. Berger, you have no idea what a relief that is. I thought I must be going crazy. You know, really losing my grip." That's little wonder, so wide is the spectrum of psychological upset PMS can cause. Wendy had always been proud of her sunny and energetic disposition. Now, at age twenty-nine, she felt herself careening on a roller coaster of binges, crying jags, and growing irritability with her young daughter, Shawna. She had finally come to me, very disturbed, because she was feeling so out of control. Afraid it might get worse, afraid she might snap and do something truly destructive, Wendy didn't know where to turn. Her regular family physician had shrugged and suggested a psychiatrist. But Wendy knew that wasn't the answer, or at least not all of it. "It's so confusing," she explained, "Most of the time, I feel great—just like myself, you know?" It was just that sometimes, on what she saw as no particular schedule, things got "all dark and crazy." Of course, when things were at their worst was exactly when Wendy could least clearly be objective and see that there was a pattern.

For Wendy, as for so many PMS patients, coming to my office was the first time they compared their shifting array of disturbing symptoms with a calendar. It is always a tremendous relief to hear, "You're not crazy, you've got PMS."

The final good reason for you to pinpoint the occurrence of your symptoms is a practical one. By knowing your PMS window, you can arrange your life to account for it, both by making life-style changes in the days before in an attempt to eliminate or minimize the PMS effects and by making sure that you don't schedule highly stressful or important events during your critical period. Obviously, this would not be the best time to be closing a delicate business negotiation, engaging in stressful interpersonal relations, or taking the final exam for your pilot's license. Knowing your own biological schedule means giving yourself an extra advantage.

## PMS Symptom Log

| DATE | PHYSICAL CONDITION/ SYMPTOM | MOOD/ EMOTION | LIFE EVENTS | CYCLE DAY |
|------|------|------|------|------|
|  |  |  |  |  |
|  |  |  |  |  |
|  |  |  |  |  |
|  |  |  |  |  |
|  |  |  |  |  |
|  |  |  |  |  |
|  |  |  |  |  |
|  |  |  |  |  |
|  |  |  |  |  |
|  |  |  |  |  |
|  |  |  |  |  |

Happily, figuring out your own window is very simple. I ask patients to take a special calendar and to chart, for three months, their mental, emotional, and physical ups and downs. On the calendar, I also ask them to note any particularly obvious life events—the death of a friend, getting a promotion at work, an impending deadline or a vacation trip—that could account for normal, non-PMS-related ups and downs.

Just how complex you want to make this calendar is up to you. I have had patients who love to go all out, using colored pens to note their moods, symptoms, and energy levels, and keeping elaborate diaries of what events and stresses were going on in their lives each day. Others prefer a more streamlined approach, simply noting a specific numeric rating for mood, physical health, and energy every day.

I use a very simple form that allows you to list both not only how you feel and the changing events of your life but also the day of your regular cycle. It appears on page 215, if you want to adapt it or use it as is to keep your own PMS log.

The exact form of your log doesn't matter so much as the fact that you mark it consistently, every day, and that you use a standardized form of notation, to make comparisons easier. Some days you may feel simply too tired, too beset, or too irritable to mark your PMS calendar. Well, that is important in itself. If you are feeling that way, there may well be a biochemical reason, and it may well be exactly the kind of information you ought to have in the log. Mark it down!

Pay particular attention to the column "Cycle Day." Here, you should mark which day of your menstrual cycle it is. True PMS symptoms follow this cycle in a characteristic pattern. The key steps are:

1. No symptoms in the week after your period
2. Gradual rise in symptoms starting from about ten days or two weeks after your period (luteal phase of cycle)

3. Most intense, disturbing symptoms in the days immediately before your period
4. Dramatic relief of symptoms when monthly bleeding occurs

When it comes to PMS, a picture is indeed worth a thousand words. This graph gives a better feeling for the typical pattern of PMS symptoms.

---

## SYMPTOMS AND PMS

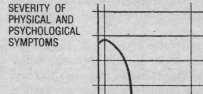
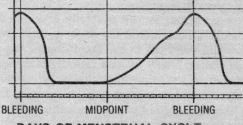

SEVERITY OF PHYSICAL AND PSYCHOLOGICAL SYMPTOMS

BLEEDING            MIDPOINT            BLEEDING

**DAYS OF MENSTRUAL CYCLE**

---

Just as the tight schedule of PMS helps you pinpoint PMS, it also helps you in another way: by possibly ruling out the syndrome. If you find that you are suffering from several of the broad constellation of PMS symptoms, *but they are not happening on the PMS schedule,* it is the best clue that you should look to other causes elsewhere. Perhaps the cause is another phantom, such as hypothyroid or hypoglycemia, or perhaps any of a range of specific medical or psychological illnesses. Clearly, though, if what you have doesn't keep the classic PMS schedule—building to a peak just before your period and diminishing rapidly thereafter—you can rule out this phantom.

## Are You a Likely PMS Victim?

So far we've seen that the "whats" don't do a very good job of defining PMS and that the "whens" are an invaluable aid to pinpointing PMS problems. But there is one other area, often overlooked, that can be helpful. That is the "whos."

The primary risk group for PMS is so obvious as to be self-evident: women from fifteen to fifty. Obviously, you can't have *pre*-menstrual symptoms without having a menstrual period! But we now know that there are other subdivisions of this rather broad category, which can tell us more about what groups may be likely to have more PMS problems than others.

For reasons we do not fully understand, PMS commonly appears not at the beginning of a woman's childbearing years but in her late twenties and early thirties. Of course, many women report PMS problems earlier, and some don't show their first symptom until many years later. But as a general rule, researchers have noticed a statistical bulge in women reporting problems in this age group.

It can be tremendously disconcerting for a woman who may have been menstruating for fifteen years to begin all of a sudden to experience the discomfort and difficulties of PMS. But she should not assume that that suggests there is something biologically awry with her body. It is just the pattern often observed with this disease, for reasons that are not yet clear.

Doctors have also noticed that the onset of PMS symptoms can often be triggered by disruptions within the female reproductive tract, such as surgical sterilization or the birth of a child.

The other quite clear group linked to PMS problems are women who consume significant amounts of caffeine. This can be a very insidious factor, because caffeine hides in so many of the substances we take into our bodies on a daily basis. It's far more than just coffee and tea. It also includes many colas, over-the-counter remedies for colds and flu, even chocolate and cocoa.

A recent report in the *American Journal of Public Health* corroborated the fact that "consumption of caffeine-containing beverages is strongly related to the presence and severity of PMS." The researcher, who studied 295 college sophomores, went on to say that the effects of caffeine seem to be linked to the whole spectrum of PMS symptoms. She cited biochemical studies suggesting that caffeine may even be an actual *cause* of PMS.

One other tantalizing study addressed the difference between those women who *have* PMS and those who *report* the most problems with it. The researchers, reporting in the *Journal of Reproductive Medicine,* found some very interesting facts about who is most vulnerable to the predations of this disease. They learned that homemakers and women with less educational and career achievement are more likely to report significant symptoms. Several factors may lie behind this interesting finding, including these women's level of general satisfaction with their lives and the degree to which their life-style distracts them from, or masks, their PMS symptoms.

## PMS Panaceas

Having looked at almost every other aspect of this puzzling syndrome, I want to close with the part that is probably the most important to you: what you can do about lessening the toll PMS takes on your life.

One recent study showed that more than a quarter of the women studied had serious enough PMS symptoms to motivate them to seek professional help. If you are one of the many women who ends up in the consulting room of a physician looking for relief, you should have at least some familiarity with what you may be offered. The most popular remedies include:

- Treatment with natural progesterone hormones, to try to regulate your hormonal balance back into steady equilibrium.
- Treatment with drugs to reduce the water gain that, some physicians believe, lies at the root of other PMS symptoms. These medications may include standard diuretics or drugs, including bromocriptine or spironolactone, which block the hormonal chain leading to water retention
- Treatment with psychoactive medications, such as antianxiety medications, tranquilizers, and the antidepressant lithium.
- Treatment with oral contraceptives to regulate the body's hormonal changes

As you can see from this list, there is no shortage of medical-pharmacological solutions that have been theorized about, tested, and tried for PMS. These approaches may seem varied and diverse, but believe me, they represent only the tiniest tip of the PMS-treatment iceberg. One researcher at Baylor Medical School reported 327 different drugs listed in the medical literature for this condition! But almost all these pharmacological (drug-based) cures seem to share one trait in common: They don't really work.

Don't just take my word for it. Listen to a cross-section of what eminent authorities have said about PMS cures:

Currently, no one can say . . . how best to treat PMS. ("The Premenstrual Enigma": *The Harvard Medical School Health Letter,* Aug. 1984, Vol. IX, No. 10, p. 1.)

No consistently effective approach has been found to help all women with PMS. (Chakmakjian, Zaren H., M.D., "Critical Assessment of Therapy for Premenstrual Tension Syndrome," *Journal of Reproductive Medicine,* Aug. 1983, Vol. 28, No. 8, p. 532.)

There is no clear-cut evidence of the effectiveness of any . . . medical approaches. (Keye, William R., M.D., "Medical Treatment of Pre-Menstrual Syndrome," *Canadian Journal of Psychiatry*, Nov. 1985, Vol. 30, p. 483.)

No single treatment is uniformly effective. ("Premenstrual Syndrome," *Mayo Clinic Health Letter*, Feb. 1987, p. 6.)

Whew—discouraging, isn't it? In a way, that's hardly surprising. After all, we have seen that PMS is certainly not a typical disease in any other sense. We can't define it, can't test for it, and can't diagnose it solely by its symptoms. Since everything else about this disease has gone against the medical grain, why should its treatment be any different?

## The Road to Holistic Health

But don't give up yet, because there are a few answers hidden in all this. All of the quotes above referred to specifically pharmacological, drug-based attempts at treatment. Yet, it turns out, in order to have a running chance at controlling this disease, we have to look beyond the confines of medicine bottles and pharmacies. For it now appears that the best hope for controlling PMS comes not from drugs at all, but from a much more holistic regimen, involving three factors: diet, vitamins, and life-style.

## Step One: Eat the Blues Away!

Although the armamentarium of drugs doesn't work very well, one thing that almost all PMS-aware doctors agree on is that dietary changes can have a significantly positive effect in most cases of PMS. A special survey of 1,600 physicians by a PMS newsletter showed that, of the doctors responding to a questionnaire, *up to 86 percent of them recommended dietary changes to their patients.*

What do all these doctors know that you don't? The basics of an anti-PMS diet can be summed up in a few simple principles:

- Reduce your intake of caffeine in all forms—coffee, tea, colas, chocolate.
- Avoid salty foods, which will aggravate a water-retention problem.
- Switch to a diet higher in protein and lower in fat, including high-protein snacks between meals.
- Reduce the amount of refined sugar in your diet, to minimize mood and energy swings.
- Reduce your intake of alcohol.
- Reduce your weight to an optimal level.
- Increase your intake of raw, unprocessed, and high-fiber foods.

You may notice something familiar about these suggestions. First, they all make good dietary sense anyway and can only help keep you healthy and energetic, regardless of whether you have PMS symptoms. Whether or not they will help in specific cases of PMS is not 100 percent clear. But what is clear is that they can't hurt—and the rules of good nutrition suggest that you should be doing them anyway!

The second fact you might note about them is that most of these counsels break down into one of two categories:

- Changes that help stabilize your mood and energy, corresponding to the attention to sugar, protein, high-fiber, alcohol, and caffeine.
- Changes that help rid your body of damaging "excess cargo," which aggravates PMS, corresponding to the tips on weight reduction and intake of salt, alcohol, and fat.

That is, they boil down to "stabilizing" and "shedding." Taken together, these two principles can really help you make a significant dent in most PMS symptoms.

## Step Two: Mind Your Micronutrients

Micronutrients—vitamins, minerals, and amino acids—each may have an important role to play in controlling PMS. The use of one vitamin, in fact—vitamin $B_6$ (also called pyridoxine)—is the second most commonly prescribed way to alleviate PMS problems. Pyridoxine has been found by several research teams to be an effective means for some women to reduce their PMS symptoms.

One study, from Britain's leading PMS center, found that 63 percent of women taking vitamin $B_6$ had a marked decrease in their PMS symptoms, as compared with a control group receiving inactive placebos.

Another research article focused specifically on the effects of $B_6$ for women suffering from the mood and emotional disturbances of PMS. The doctors found that the vitamin reduced or eliminated symptoms of depression, fatigue, mild paranoia, and difficulty concentrating for three-quarters of the women.

One final study, reported from Scotland, showed that women receiving $B_6$ supplements were three times more likely to report improvements in their health than women taking placebos and that no side effects were reported.

In fact, the side-effects issue is not quite so clear-cut as all that. Our own *New England Journal of Medicine* reports that women taking too much $B_6$ can start to experience serious neurological symptoms, including numbness and tingling of the extremities. The good news, however, is that such symptoms only seem to happen when women take far too much of the vitamin. (Some had taken up to a hundred times the recommended dose!)

But at normal levels, the vitamin is well tolerated, inexpensive, and has no side effects. With that in mind, you should keep your $B_6$ dose at the levels used by research scientists: no more than 100 milligrams daily, taken only for the ten days prior to menstruation. It is not necessary, or even helpful, to continue taking such high levels of the vitamin the rest of the month. I suggest to my patients that they take their $B_6$ in the morning, to make sure that it is optimally absorbed and that it does not interfere with sleep.

In addition to vitamin $B_6$, the micronutrient mineral magnesium may also play an important role in helping you overcome a wide range of PMS problems. Several research papers suggest that magnesium has been found useful by doctors in treating PMS. Although there have been few well-controlled studies, and there clearly remains much we have to learn about this nutrient and PMS, it also seems clear that it can be a helpful link in a chain to help you pull yourself out of the PMS pit.

Because magnesium is a vital micromineral for many of the body's systems—including your heart and muscles—it is a good idea on general principles to get enough of it. But some people, especially those with heart or kidney problems, can run into trouble taking this mineral. For that reason, I suggest that you consult your doctor before taking any magnesium supplements for PMS.

But what you can do, without any doctor's help, is to make sure that you are eating foods that are naturally rich in this health-giving mineral. These include green leafy vegetables, seafood, nuts, cereal, grains, and dairy products. By eating a diet rich in these basic elements you will help replenish your body's magnesium stores, another key element in the PMS battle.

The final micronutrient you should know about is the amino acid L-tryptophan. Research from the Premenstrual Solution, a help and resource organization for PMS sufferers, shows that this amino acid can have a significant effect to minimize PMS symptoms of anger, crying spells, irritability, depression, and mood swings. This amino acid is one of the building blocks of full proteins. As a naturally occurring amino acid, it is found in significant quantities in foods such as yogurt, pineapple, and turkey. Biochemically, the tryptophan you eat is converted in your brain to the crucial neurotransmitter serotonin, which helps your brain regulate sleep patterns and emotional stability.

While we do not understand all the details of the tryptophan-PMS link, studies show that women taking up to 1,500 milligrams daily experience relief from PMS symptoms. I recommend to some of my PMS patients that they take 500 milligrams each day—250 milligrams during the daytime and another 250 milligrams about a half hour before going to sleep. This works as a safe, natural sleep inducer and seems to help regulate their sleep and emotional cycles.

Of course, if you are interested in using tryptophan, I suggest you do so in cooperation with your own physician, so that he or she can help integrate this into an overall PMS plan that works for you.

## Step Three: Build a PMS-Proof Life-Style

The third step in making yourself "PMS-proof" involves changes in your life-style in two primary areas: stress and exercise.

The first, stress, is fairly obvious. Because PMS seems so clearly linked to a disruption of the body's normal balance of systems, it makes sense that you don't want to do anything to further throw off your biological equilibrium. Stress of all kinds—personal, physical, emotional, or career—does exactly that. The moral is simple: avoiding extra stresses in your vulnerable "PMS window" may pay off in fewer, shorter, and less severe PMS symptoms.

Of course, in most of our frenetic, pressured, fast-paced lives, avoiding stress is more easily said than done. But sometimes stressful living is more of a necessity than it is a destructive habit. If that might be the case for you, I suggest you keep in mind three simple ways to reduce stress:

1. *Allow yourself to say no.* Many of the demands made on you can just as easily be done by someone else—or by you at some other time. That extra car pool trip, the "just this once" favor for a friend, the rush job at the office, entertaining the boss at home—all are extra sources of tension and pressure. I am not saying you can never do them, but that, surprisingly often, you can say no—at least until you are out of your PMS danger window. Then feel free to take on the extras, with the confidence that you'll do them better and more efficiently now that you're out of your PMS window.

2. *Sleep.* As Shakespeare wrote, sleep knits the raveled sleeve of care. I doubt that he had PMS on his mind at the time, but the wisdom holds true. Sleep may be your single biggest ally in building your body's strength and resiliency in your PMS window. That is just the time to forget those midweek late-night soirees and avoid scheduling social or work entanglements that deprive you of much-needed pillow time. Chances are this is exactly when your body will naturally be craving more sleep, anyway, so you should indulge it. You—and your family, mate, and co-workers—will be glad you did! (Then, the rest of the month, you can socialize to your heart's content!)

3. *Take some time for yourself.* Each of us has ways of reducing our stress load. Maybe for you, it's playing the piano, writing to friends, weeding the garden, or curling up with a good book in a quiet room. Whatever is the special activity that makes you feel pampered, now's the time to make sure you do it. You don't have to make a major production out of it, but just take the time you need to give yourself an island of tranquillity in the midst of your tempestuous days. Five or ten minutes may well be enough, just so long as *you* feel you have had a breather. Consider it a dose of preventive medicine against PMS. If anybody asks what you're doing, well, tell them you're simply following orders from Dr. Berger.

## Get Exercised!

That may not make much sense, especially after what I just said about reducing tension. But I don't mean the kind of exercise where you rant and rave and shout. I mean the kind where you huff and puff and sweat. Specifically, aerobic exercise, about twenty minutes each day.

Physicians now think that exercise works to reduce PMS problems in several ways. First of all, it helps your body lose excess fluid and burn off excess fat, both of which help PMS. By reducing fat, it also lowers the amount of the female hormone estrogen your body produces. In these three ways, it seems to "turn down" the biochemical *Sturm und Drang* that underlies PMS.

Exercise helps in another way, too. Biochemically, it increases the level of endorphins, your body's "natural opiates." These chemicals help you feel more tranquil, improve your ability to tolerate stress, even soothe the minor aches and pains that PMS can bring. It's like giving yourself a natural high, one that protects against PMS, and the best way to do it is by exercise.

The final way exercise helps is that it stretches and warms up your muscles. If you are tense with PMS stress, it is a fair bet that one of the first places that tension settles is in your muscles. Exercise gives you a chance to flush that tension out of your muscles, and so out of your body.

So much for the theory of it all. Does it work? Yes, says a study of 748 Finnish women. Researchers found that women who regularly participated in sports reported significantly less premenstrual anxiety than a matched group of women who didn't get such exercise. Anecdotal evidence from women athletes in this country shows much the same thing—that moderate, steady exercise helps keep the phantom of PMS at bay.

Note, though, the key word *moderate*. If you exercise too hard, you may actually disrupt your menstrual cycle and become amenorrheic. This is fairly commonly noted with women who exercise too strenuously, in athletics, running, or weight lifting. You don't want to go this far, since such a disruption can have less-than-healthy effects all throughout your endocrine (hormonal) system.

When it comes to exercise for PMS, the best prescription is the one the Greeks knew about long ago: the golden mean, moderation. In your own life that translates to moderate aerobic exercise every day or at least several times a week. Try it for a month, and you'll be amazed at how much better you look, feel, and act!

## In a Nutshell . . .

To sum up, it may help to remember the changes that are under your control that can help you fight the phantom of PMS:

1. *Diet*
   Reduce caffeine
   Avoid salty foods
   Increase protein, reduce fat
   Reduce refined sugar
   Reduce alcohol
   Reduce your weight
   Eat more raw, high-fiber foods
2. *Nutrient Supplements*
   Take 100 milligrams of vitamin $B_6$ (pyridoxine) daily
   Eat magnesium-rich foods
   Take up to 500 milligrams of L-tryptophan amino acid
3. *Stress Management and Exercise*
   Learn to say no
   Get enough sleep
   Take time for yourself
   Get twenty minutes of aerobic exercise several times each week

If you make these changes and still have problems, you may want to consult your physician, who may recommend a drug treatment. But before you do that, I hope you'll give a fair try to all these changes that you can make on your own.

## Get Thee Behind Me, Phantom

What I hope this chapter has given you is a good overview of the important aspects of premenstrual syndrome. Together, we have examined its symptoms and highly specific schedule and seen the damage it can cause and how it is so often ignored and overlooked by the conventional medical wisdom.

But more important, you have seen the many ways you can take steps in your own life, in a cooperative, mutually supportive relationship with your own doctor, to make PMS a problem in your past.

To be sure, that will require some work on your part: careful observation of your symptoms and emotions, conscientious diary keeping, and devoted attention to factors such as diet and life-style. But if you do that, I can almost guarantee that you will look, act, and feel better and that you can put these "once-a-month-beastlies" behind you once and for all. Once you do that, you'll wonder why you waited so long to do it!

## For Deeper Study

*PMS Access.* P.O. Box 9326, Madison, Wisconsin. Tel. (800) 222-4PMS; in Wisconsin (608) 833-4PMS. This bimonthly newsletter is a valuable source of information for PMS sufferers.

Michelle Harrison, M.D., *Self-Help for Premenstrual Syndrome.* New York: Random House, 1985.

*The Premenstrual Solution.* 1833 Farndon Avenue, Los Altos, California 94022. Tel. (415) 961-9430.

# 12

# The Virulent Viruses:
# A Trio of Phantoms

It is a phenomenon that occurs only rarely in medical history: the birth of a disease. Unfortunately, in our generation we have witnessed the uncovering of one of the most chilling examples of a new disease in recent world history, AIDS. Ten years ago this disease had never been seen in humans. Then, because of a chance, random mutation of a virus, it sprang into existence—virulent, full blown, and deadly. Today we watch helplessly as this infectious newcomer casts its tragic shadow across our entire globe.

This chapter is not concerned with AIDS, for it is not a phantom. (It is, in fact, the furthest thing from a true phantom. Not only has it been the subject of intense public attention, glaring media coverage, and profound scientific scrutiny, but its symptoms are usually rather clear and distinctive, its diagnosis agreed on and relatively straightforward.)

But although the phantoms I want to discuss in this chapter are not AIDS, they do share several traits with that disease. Like AIDS, they have come into public recognition very recently—98 percent of the research papers about these viral diseases have been published in the last four years. One of these viral suspects is so new, in fact, that it was not even discovered until late last year! Like AIDS, they, too, are caused by inestimably small, spherical viruses, members of the herpesvirus family. Like the AIDS virus, these phantom viruses can harbor themselves in your body in a dormant or latent phase, often for many years, before they get reactivated, making you sick with a variety of debilitating, systemic symptoms. Finally, like AIDS, the first of these viruses I want to explore has been christened with a four-letter medical acronym: CEBV, or chronic Epstein-Barr virus.

Fortunately, though, this phantom does not mirror AIDS in every particular. For CEBV is not a killer. Instead, it does its damage by giving you a protracted low-level illness, profoundly undermining your energy and vitality. CEBV victims find themselves overcome by relentless, overwhelming fatigue. They are left depressed, depleted, and sickly, sometimes for several years at a time. There are even cases where doctors report these viral infections apparently lasting twenty, thirty, even forty years! Imagine a disease that can submerge half an entire lifetime in a dreary fog of depression, sluggishness, lost opportunity, and sapped vitality, and you begin to understand the destructive power of this viral phantom.

## Don't *You* Be a Viral Victim!

CEBV and its virus cousins bear all the markings of classic phantoms. It is newly arrived, and underrecognized, and it brings with it a range of tremendous, debilitating health problems. Most important of all, perhaps more than with any of the other phantoms we have seen, there is a very good chance a practicing physician can miss its diagnosis. With qualities like that, it is doubly important that *you* understand what we do know about it—so that you and your loved ones can avoid becoming "viral victims."

## The Nevada Virus—An Epidemic Is Born

The sleepy town of Incline Village is an unlikely place for medical history to unfold. Situated on the shores of Lake Tahoe in the spectacularly beautiful Sierra Nevada mountains, it is the kind of place where people go to escape the drama of modern living. But starting in the fall of 1984, something very ominous was happening to the 4,000 residents of this Nevada town. Two local doctors noticed that their patients were suddenly coming in with many of the same complaints: profound fatigue; prolonged sore throat; swollen glands, spleen, or liver. At first there was little alarm. Many of these were the symptoms of a regular flu germ, the kind that usually persist for ten days or two weeks, then go away. But in tranquil Incline Village, there was one crucial difference: It wasn't going away. It dragged on, debilitating people for weeks, even months. Too, the physicians noted, there were many people who complained of tremendous, disabling fatigue. Over the winter months the numbers mounted, and soon the town had more than 130 people with these same inexplicable fatigue symptoms.

Puzzled, the doctors tested their sick patients' blood— and found in many of them surprisingly elevated levels of Epstein-Barr virus (EBV) antibodies, a profile highly suggestive of an active EBV infection. Alarmed and curious, epidemiological experts from the Centers for Disease Control soon swarmed to the area to investigate the outbreak and look at the EBV connection.

At that time, doctors were already quite familiar with EBV. The virus had been discovered in 1964, twenty years before the mysterious flu outbreak in Nevada. We already knew that EBV played a role in several conditions. Most commonly, in this country, it is known as the agent behind infectious mononucleosis, the "kissing disease" that is so common among adolescents and young adults. EBV, the experts knew, could make you sick, even overwhelmingly exhausted, for several weeks or months—but then it goes away. EBV had also been associated with two uncommon forms of cancer: one, occurring mainly in equatorial Africa, another a cancer of the nasal tract that is rare in this country—both somewhat esoteric footnotes of medical textbooks. But except for those uncommon exceptions, the medical establishment thought it largely understood the *modus operandi* of this viral marauder.

As things turned out, the medical establishment was wrong. What we have learned in the last several years—and what the Nevada epidemic was further to suggest—was that this old virus has a more serious face.

By a quirk of medical happenstance, two research papers appeared in the *Annals of Internal Medicine* just a few months before the epidemic hit Incline Village. They held tantalizing clues, suggesting that plain Epstein-Barr virus might have a long-lasting alter ego, that sometimes it doesn't just go away, but lingers on. The possibility had been hanging around in corners of the medical community since it was first reported in the 1960s. But here, suddenly, was the kind of conjunction that makes medical history. These papers, combined with earlier journal articles, made the medical community begin to wonder if this might have something to do with the mysterious epidemic of endless flu in Incline Village. As we understood that Epstein-Barr virus could become *chronic* Epstein-Barr virus, the *C* was added to the acronym, and the phantom was born.

Today our whole scientific conception of this virus is being radically overhauled. Leading virologists, epidemiologists, and physicians are engaged in exhaustive research to help track down this most exhausting virus. As I write this, they are holding a series of meetings to redefine what we know about this viral syndrome, and the Centers for Disease Control is trying to come up with a solid, clinical definition of the syndrome.

The Incline Village epidemic remains an unsolved medical detective story, a scientific work in progress. The team of experts were never able to prove conclusively the EBV was the cause of the epidemic, but they were not able to exonerate it either. What they found was a suggestive trail of clues and biological hints hidden in the blood of those victims, suggesting that EBV played some central role in the drama. Ironically, we may never know what happened in Incline Village, but the spotlight it put on EBV has made real scientific headlines. What they unearthed has real implications for you, your family, and every American.

For one thing, it has suggested a possible explanation for a rash of other such outbreaks. In the last half century, there have been some thirty other such mysterious epidemics. They have been called different things at different times—Iceland disease, Akureyri disease, Royal Free disease, and benign myalgic encephalomyelitis are just a few of them—but the symptoms are remarkably similar, including fatigue, headache, weakness, and depression. All bore a suspicious resemblance to what happened in Incline Village.

For the people of that mountain hamlet, there was little to do but to continue fighting the disease that had attacked them. After several months, many of them got better as the virus seemed to mysteriously go away, back to wherever it came from. But for some, the story was not over. Today, more than two years later, many of the sick Incline Village residents are still too tired to return to their lives and jobs.

Yet for the scientific community, and ultimately for you, the episode helped open a whole new door. What began as a rare and serendipitous coincidence between clinical research and a quiet mountain hamlet has given us a new look at an old virus. Through it, we have now found ourselves facing a brand-new phantom head-on.

Researchers now believe the CEBV is only part of the answer to this disease riddle. There are other viruses, in the same viral family, which I will discuss later in this chapter. The more we learn, the more we think that they, too, play a role in these mysterious and crippling viral syndromes. But first, let's look at the vital CEBV connection and what it may mean for you.

## A Virus by Any Other Name

The more research that is done in this area, the more convincing grows the case: Many, many Americans have suffered from—or are now in the grip of—a viral disease syndrome that, until now, we have had no name for.

We have recognized the problem so recently, in fact, that medical experts have yet to make up their minds completely about what to call it. Some scientists term the problem *chronic mononucleosis* or *recurrent mononucleosis*, drawing a link between this and the short-term disease usually caused by EBV. Researchers at the Centers for Disease Control, in Atlanta, have coined the term *mononucleosis-like syndrome*. Others, recognizing important differences between the short- and long-term versions, term it *chronic Epstein-Barr virus*, or *CEBV*—the term I prefer. Still others use the catchall label *neuromyasthenia*, a loosely defined medical term meaning profound weakness of nerves and muscles, often with depression and headaches.

It may take years before we agree just what to call it, but that hardly matters. What is clear, from researchers around the world, is that this phantom is very real:

• A group of Israeli physicians followed seven patients with vague symptoms, including fatigue, swollen glands, weakness, and fevers. All of the patients were found to have high levels of antibodies to EBV in their blood, suggesting that their bodies were trying to fight off the virus.

• A pivotal study, published in the *Annals of Internal Medicine*, examined a group of adults and children suffering from a mysterious, long-term sickness. Their symptoms: tremendous fatigue, depression, sore throats and joint pain, headaches, fever, and swollen glands. When the doctors tested them for antibodies to EB virus, they found that almost 90 percent of them had "antibody levels compatible with active infection for *at least one year*. (emphasis added)

• Scientists at the National Institute of Allergy and Infectious Diseases examined thirty-one patients who had been referred to them suffering from chronic, debilitating fatigue diseases that had lasted at least eighteen months (in some cases up to five years). Fully half of the patients had such serious malaise that they could not work. In fully 74 percent of them—almost three-quarters—blood tests suggested that undiagnosed CEBV was the likely culprit.

• Writing in the *Canadian Medical Association Journal,* a physician examined fifty patients suffering from "prolonged and excessive fatigue." Among those who could be successfully diagnosed, the single largest group was those suffering from apparent viral diseases, accounting for about half of the cases. Of those, 70 percent were found to have the chronic form of Epstein-Barr virus—the CEBV phantom.

The research breakthroughs from these sources brings tremendously hopeful news to a lot of long-suffering people. To find out if you are one of them, read the next pages carefully!

## New Research, New Hope

The simple truth is that we do not know how many people have this disease, because relatively few physicians have started looking for it in any informed, systematic way. But the estimates range in the tens of thousands in this country alone, according to experts.

Clearly, these researchers' "early returns" suggest that we are seeing only the beginning of this phantom. In the time since the news has begun to be disseminated in the scientific and medical community, researchers at the National Institutes of Health have been flooded with letters from people reporting the viral syndrome of CEBV. In just two years, the National CEBV Syndrome Association, a national clearinghouse for CEBV sufferers, already counts some twelve thousand members in its ranks, and its president estimates there are "tens of thousands" more nationwide. So many people are concerned that they may

## EPSTEIN-BARR VIRUS

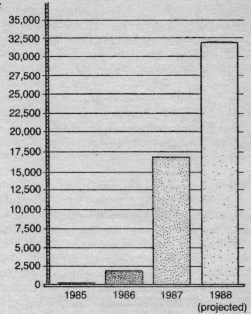

**NUMBER OF CEBV CASES REPORTED**

*Source: CEBV Association*

be affected that self-help groups have formed in a score of cities here, and in several countries abroad, to counsel CEBV viral syndrome sufferers.

Now, medical experts are not soothsayers, and we cannot foretell the future. But it is clear that as physicians practicing in the front lines of medicine learn more about CEBV, we can expect the number of reported cases to swell dramatically. If we are to judge by the pattern over the last few years, it doesn't take much imagination to predict what the trajectory of this particular phantom could look like.

## The Path of a Phantom

Of course, it really doesn't matter whether this phantom affects ten thousand or ten times that number. That is just the medical numbers game. What matters is the very real, and very insidious, possibility that you or your mate, family, or friends might find yourself among them.

## Death, Taxes, and EBV

*"Epstein-Barr viral infection, like death and taxes, is virtually inevitable among humans."*
Journal of Human Pathology

One of the reasons that this disease has the potential to be so widespread is that, in one way, we all already have it. Or, to be more precise, although you may not necessarily have the disease, you have the virus that causes it.

Like the *Candida* yeast organisms we met earlier, this virus lives full-time in almost all of us. You are exposed to it throughout your life, and by the time you reached age ten, you already had about a fifty-fifty chance of already having this virus as a full-time resident in your body. If you have reached middle adulthood, your odds are virtually 100 percent that you harbor EB virus. (If that idea bothers you, I suggest that you can take comfort in one simple fact. If you lived in most other less-developed countries of the world, you would not even have escaped early childhood without a 100 percent probability of contracting the virus.)

This helps explain why we often get "mono" in adolescence and early adulthood. You might say it represents a viral marker for "coming of age." Studies have shown that only half of the teenagers entering college—a group, for the most part, of clear economic, and health, privilege—have encountered EBV yet. Not surprisingly, when such people, protected from infection by the virus so far, encounter it as an adult, they get noticeably sicker than if they had contracted the disease as a child. The same bug that might have passed unnoticed, or as a minor flulike bug, at age eight, becomes more important at age eighteen. About a third of those who encounter EBV during these years will come down with a disease serious enough to be diagnosed as infectious mononucleosis.

Once you have the virus inside you, you become part of the "problem." The virus rides around in your body, secreted inside a special kind of white blood cell, your B lymphocytes. If it only behaved itself and stayed put, it would be less of a problem. But it doesn't. In one person out of five, the virus gets into the saliva, and from there you can transmit it to the outside world—and spread EBV further. Because this virus is so easily transmitted (unlike, say, the AIDS virus, which is not transmitted by saliva), it is no surprise that almost everybody in the world, by the age of thirty or so, is an EBV carrier.

So why aren't we all sick all the time? Simple. The virus, like other members of the herpesvirus family, goes into a latent phase. Like a bear hibernating in its winter's den, the virus curls up in your B cells and does the viral equivalent of "a long winter's nap." With luck, it will never wake up—what scientists term *reactivation*. Or, if and when it does, you might come down with classic, short-term mononucleosis, then rebound. But a small, unlucky percentage go down another road. They come down with the same monolike illness, but do not fight it off. Instead, their EBV infection "goes chronic," and they find themselves caught in the tenacious grip of this phantom, paying the price in sapped energy, lost vitality, and diminished health. Others may not even suffer the acute phase of the illness at all, but simply start sliding down into an insidious cycle of diminished energy, vitality, and health.

That is what happened to Susan T. She was the classic overachiever. By age thirty-two she had won a high-powered job as a regional vice president for a major financial services firm. Her life seemed ideal until about three years ago, when her father died unexpectedly. Although Susan's whole family was numbed by the sudden shock and grief, for her, it affected her health. During the next flu season, it seemed as though she was constantly sick with one flu or another. As spring came, she expected that the rash of illness would abate, but it didn't. Instead, she became seriously exhausted.

Determining something had to be done, Susan saw her doctor, a woman she had seen for years and trusted completely. After weeks of tests, the doctor could find nothing "really wrong," said she was undoubtedly working too hard, and prescribed rest.

"That was true, as far as it went," recalls Susan. Yes, there had been a lot of stress at the office, new managers, changes, and a plethora of new responsibilities. "But I knew that wasn't it. Work had always been incredibly hectic. That was no different than ever. What was different was me. I was just completely burned out." Discouraged, she went to two other doctors, neither of whom could offer anything.

The summer passed, and as her friends and associates played, Susan only got worse. The fatigue was all but overwhelming. At work, she was clearly in some trouble. Her fatigue made it impossible to really concentrate. Her keen mind—the prime requisite for her intellectually demanding, fast-paced job—seemed dulled and fuzzy. Each day she dragged herself home from the office with barely enough energy to fall into bed, sometimes without even eating dinner. Her afterwork life, once a whirlwind of professional and social commitments, dwindled to a trickle, then stopped altogether as she had to husband her energy for herself. Even her closest friends began to drift away. It was, in Susan's words, as though "all the lights in my world were blinking off, one by one. And there was nothing I could do about it. I just didn't care anymore."

When I saw Susan, I ran the usual tests that the other doctors had run. Finding nothing, I turned to the possibility of CEBV—and hit pay dirt. Her blood tests revealed the particular antibody profile consistent with active EBV infection. That is not necessarily definitive (you'll see why, soon) but in combination with Susan's life-wrenching symptoms, I suspected we had found her phantom.

But that was only half the battle. With many of the phantoms we have seen, including *Candida*, hypothyroid, labile hypertension, and silent ischemia, the real challenge is tracking them down in the first place. After that, treatment is often relatively straightforward. Unfortunately, I had to tell Susan that with CBV, the next step is not nearly so simple. I prescribed a strong immune-boosting regimen, based on the formula I developed in *Dr. Berger's Immune Power Diet,* which has worked for thousands of people. It incorporated a plan of vitamins, minerals, and amino acids and removed specific foods that could be causing Susan allergy problems. The goal, as I explained to her, was to rebuild her body's own immune competence, so it could fight her EB virus back into dormancy.

As she left that day, she smiled wearily. "You have no idea how much better I feel already, Dr. Berger. Just knowing there's a name for what I have, that I am not crazy, and that it won't get worse and worse until I shrivel away into nothing. That's a huge help."

Susan will never know just what caused the reactivation of her latent EB virus and pushed her over the brink into a chronic viral infection. It may have been the cumulative stress of her job, perhaps another viral infection, an environmental toxin, or any of hundreds of other possibilities. She only knows that she was one of the luck cases—her trial-by-virus lasted a little over fourteen months from beginning to end.

The last time I saw her, she told me her energy had returned—not all the way, but mostly. Now she was trying to pick up the pieces of her shattered life, getting used to the wonderful sensation of feeling strong and healthy again, experiencing and savoring the strength and vigor that all of us take for granted.

## The Kiss of Fatigue

Clearly, we have a lot to learn about this disease, but the thing that will be most helpful to *you* is knowing its range of symptoms. Happily, the most likely symptoms of CEBV are quite well established.

*If you have CEBV, you will almost certainly be suffering from incredible, disabling fatigue.* Believe me, I'm not just talking about "tired" here. This is absolutely, stuffing-knocked-out, weak-kneed, sleep-eighteen-hours-a-day, utter and absolute *exhaustion.*

I doubt that anyone who has not been through this can fully appreciate how profoundly and utterly exhausting CEBV can be. It has been said, by a pathologist who has studied the viral syndrome, that the English language simply has no adequate word for the tiredness CEBV sufferers endure. As I explain it to my patients, all of us know what it is like to have a bad flu, how you literally can't muster the energy to even get out of bed. Well, imagine feeling that way, day in and day out, for several months, years, *or even decades!* In one recent study, the disease lasted for a mean time of more than two years, and the proportion of time lost from daily activities, such as school and work, was almost 40 percent. Only when you hear accounts like this can you get a true feeling for the deep personal tragedy that this phantom can bring.

Some patients have asked me how they can know if the lethargy they feel could be related to a chronic viral infection, perhaps CEBV, or whether they are just simply tired. To start with, I suggest you take this simple quiz:

## Fatigue Factors

|  | Yes | No |
|---|---|---|
| 1. Is your tiredness not helped very much by sleeping (taking a weekend to catch up on sleep, naps, going to bed early for a week)? | —— | —— |
| 2. Can you pinpoint the specific time your energy level began to drop off? | —— | —— |
| 3. Do you find yourself having to curtail your normal daily activities? | —— | —— |
| 4. Are you having problems functioning at work? | —— | —— |
| 5. Did fatigue seem to come on in conjunction with other symptoms—swollen glands, sore throat, body or joint aches? | —— | —— |
| 6. Have friends, family, or co-workers commented on your tiredness? | —— | —— |

If you have several yes answers, the fatigue you are feeling may be of the extraordinary, virally related type.

Tiredness is the most obvious symptom of the CEBV phantom, but it is not the only one. Other common physical symptoms include:

Sore throat
Headache
Low, chronic fever (less than 100 degrees)
Swollen glands (especially in your neck)
Muscle and joint pains

Nor do I want to suggest that this phantom's damage is limited purely to physical symptoms. It can also take a significant and profound toll on your emotional, mental, and psychological strength. The medical literature reports that CEBV sufferers experience depression, confusion, difficulty concentrating, and problems with short-term memory. In fact, these "softer" psychological symptoms are

## CEBV SYMPTOMS

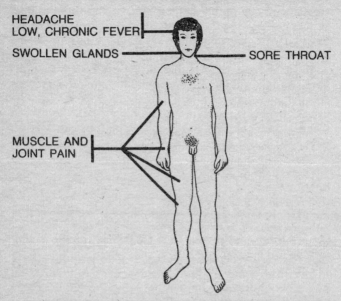

HEADACHE
LOW, CHRONIC FEVER

SWOLLEN GLANDS

SORE THROAT

MUSCLE AND
JOINT PAIN

often some of the most difficult aspects for CEBV victims to bear and are often the reasons they seek help.

The link between CEBV and depression has grown clearer just recently. In research presented at the American Psychiatric Association in its recent annual meeting, Dr. Ferris Pitts from the University of Southern California revealed that he had studied two hundred people suffering major depression. An incredible *98 percent* of them showed a distinctive antibody pattern in their blood—a pattern typical of that produced when a person is first infected with CEBV. He proposed that these depressed patients may actually be chronically fighting off a systemic virus infection, and that may be a clue to their depression.

Next, to firm up the link further, researchers looked at the problem the other way around. This time, they examined the blood of three hundred confirmed CEBV sufferers. Again, a whopping 95 percent of them had the same typical antibody profile in their blood. These studies lend further credence to the hypothesis that many cases of depression of unknown cause may actually be due to the destructive Epstein-Barr virus.

You may have noticed that all these CEBV symptoms have one major thing in common: They are all very nonspecific and general. Each of these symptoms can be caused by many, many other problems. You have seen many of them already linked to one of the phantoms we have met in earlier chapters. That is not surprising. Because CEBV infects the body's B immune cells, it sits at the center of some of our most crucial biological crossroads. From there it can easily affect your health, vitality, and mental functions.

## Doctors and CEBV: A Long Way to Go

It is this very generality that makes it so easy for CEBV to hide from doctors. Most of them aren't used to thinking of CEBV as a possible culprit for such symptoms. One Epstein-Barr sufferer who heads a chapter of the national CEBV organization has put it rather bluntly: "The majority of doctors out there don't know about this."

Just how far we have to go was made obvious in an editorial in the *Journal of the American Medical Association*. There, one of the nation's leading CEBV authorities wrote, "It no longer seems appropriate to consider all patients with the chronic fatigue symptoms to be suffering from purely psychoneurotic disorders." Imagine—the medical establishment is finally ready, in 1987, to admit that "these people aren't crazy . . . maybe they're sick after all." (The name of the article, incidentally, was "EB or Not EB—That Is the Question.")

When we hear such a sentiment just now being voiced, when we hear such timidity about recognizing a disease that is clearly taking a huge toll on so many people, you begin to see why I feel we have a very long way to go. I should say, by the way, that the author of the paper is one of the nation's preeminent CEBV researchers. If such a doctor, who has seen so many of these cases, is only just now reminding his colleagues that, indeed, something is amiss here, one can't help but realize that the average general practitioner may need some educating on the issue.

Another professional publication, *Medical World News*, recently printed the words of another doctor who has seen many CEBV patients. "Some doctors react so violently . . . they tell patients there's no such thing or say they don't believe in it" (Richard Trubo, "Viruses, the Lurking Menace," May 12, 1986, p. 56). Now of course, no self-respecting doctor would claim not to "believe in" cancer, or chicken pox. But in the case of this elusive, newborn phantom, the controversy continues, because not all physicians have yet made its acquaintance.

What that means to you is clear. It is all too easy for you to get caught in the middle. Often people are doomed to a frustrating, costly, round-robin of specialists, vainly trying to track down the phantom they know haunts them. One physician, himself knowledgeable in the ways of CEBV, reported that one patient had consulted a total of 292 different doctors over forty years of suffering! While this must be some kind of record, I know from listening to my own patients that they have often seen a score of doctors before they get to my office. Each one of them usually pronounced the problem "all in your head." (Does this sound familiar to you?)

Even the most staid medical journals have begun to recognize that most practitioners have a long way to go with CEBV. To quote from one, the *Annals of Internal Medicine*, "These patients tend to go from physician to physician in search of diagnosis and treatment." Belatedly, the medical establishment is beginning to wake up and ask if it is doing the right thing for its CEBV victims—and if not, how to improve.

Because its symptoms are so general, the best way to diagnose CEBV is by exclusion—ruling out the many other factors and illnesses that could cause the same symptoms. In real life, this is what happens most of the time, in one way or another. Usually, by the time somebody finally runs the complete blood test profiles needed to find or rule out CEBV, the patient has consulted so many doctors and endured so many tests that a whole list of other possible diagnoses has been ruled out. (Now that you have gained expertise in the phantoms, you can help short-circuit that process, by making sure your doctor is leaving no stone unturned in the search for the cause of your symptoms!)

## Are You at Risk?

Before we get to the actual nitty-gritty of the diagnostic details, it's worth taking a quick look at whether you fall into the prime-risk groups for CEBV. For reasons we do not yet understand, CEBV chooses its victims selectively. Do you fall into any of the following categories?

• Female
• Age thirty or over
• Unmarried
• College graduate
• In a high-achievement, stressful occupation
• Previously diagnosed with mononucleosis
• History of allergy, hay fever, asthma, or skin rashes

Women are up to three times more likely than men to suffer from CEBV. This is a particularly galling medical irony, of course, because women are far more likely to be dismissed as hysterical, neurotic, or hypochondriacal, particularly by the two-thirds of the physicians who are men. During the course of writing this book, I wondered more than once if the reason the medical profession is so much more likely to pigeonhole women as hypochondriacs is simply that women are more prone to the many very subtle phantom illnesses, from hypothyroidism to PMS to CEBV, diseases that men are biologically simply less likely to get.

Some of the other risk factors are a lot less clear-cut. The EB virus doesn't care, for example, that you went to college, hold a high-powered job, or aren't married (any more than the AIDS virus cares if you are gay). But still, this profile of high-achieving, white-collar CEBV sufferers seems surprisingly constant across different groups studied. (One article even dubbed it the Yuppie Flu.)

So how do we explain such a distinctive profile? In several ways. Some researchers have suggested that many normally functioning people get EBV, but they just aren't as bothered by it, because they are not used to being superachievers. Hence, it may not make such a major difference in their lives, and they may not go see a doctor about it. Or it may be that something in their life-style—the level of job-related stress or nutritional factors—may predispose this group to coming down with viral infections that, in others, would have stayed dormant.

My own view is that the pattern we are seeing here almost certainly tells us more about our medical establishment than it does about the EB virus. Such high-functioning achievers are not necessarily more likely to have CEBV, but they are more likely to be more educated and aware of their health, better able to afford to consult several doctors, more willing to buck a medical system that assures them "there's nothing wrong," and better able to eventually get themselves taken seriously by the medical profession. I think most authorities would agree that as practicing doctors learn more about CEBV, we will realize that the exclusive profile we have seen so far is really only the tip of the viral-syndrome iceberg.

The other part of the profile that is fairly clear is that this disease tends to appear most frequently in the fourth decade of life, after age thirty. There are certainly cases in adolescents and the elderly, but the bulk of them happen in the years between twenty-eight and forty-two.

As to the mono connection, it is by no means absolute. But researchers suggest that if you have previously had either mono or some undiagnosed monolike illness, you are definitely at higher risk for CEBV. It seems that between a half and a third of people with CEBV report a bout of such an illness, often in their twenties. Remember, though, this is only a risk-group predictor and not an airtight guarantee. Without having ever had mono, you can still come down with the long-lasting viral syndrome, and about a third of CEBV victims report no known previous experience with the viral disease.

Because we still have so much to learn about what these risk groups really mean, you may wonder what they have to do with you and how you can use them in your own life. I wish I could be more concrete, but I can't, because we are still too ignorant in our understanding of CEBV to put it all into perspective. What I can do is give you the same advice I give my own patients. *If* . . .

You clearly have symptoms suggesting CEBV *and*
You fit into the above risk groups *and*
Your doctor has been unable to explain your fatigue and
   other symptoms

. . . *then* you ought to make sure to discuss the possibility of CEBV with your physician. Most likely, your own doctor will be interested to find out more (believe me, there is a chance you will have more up-to-date information than some practitioners). That's perfectly okay, because I have included the "For Deeper Study" section at the end of this chapter. There you will find suggestions for further reading material for you and your doctor. If, however, you visit a practitioner who dismisses your symptoms or doesn't seem to take seriously the possible viral-CEBV connection, you may want to use the resources in that section to find a CEBV-aware doctor in your area.

## Next Step: Answers in Your Blood

Once you and your doctor have agreed to look for CEBV, the next step is quite clearly a blood test. However, this is a bit more complex than it might appear, because there really is no one simple CEBV blood test. Or, to be more accurate, there are several, and they have to be done in conjunction, and interpreted together for them to have much meaning.

You recall I said that 100 percent of adults have EBV antibodies. Obviously, then, the most direct approach—just screening for these antibodies—is not terribly useful. For by doing so, everybody who took the test would test positive! (This might be a great deal for the testing laboratories, but hardly helpful for you!)

Next it was thought that you could detect people with CEBV, because the levels of EBV antibody in their blood are much higher than the usual "background" levels most of us carry around—up to one hundred times higher. To do that, some physicians gave the standard, first-line tests for EBV antibody, called VCA-IgG. If you showed a certain level, it could suggest that the root of your problems was a CEBV infection.

But new research shows that these levels are extremely variable. Robustly healthy and energetic people can have higher levels of the antibody than some people who have the symptoms of CEBV. Another study showed that more than 10 percent of people who had had infectious mono several years before retained high levels of certain EBV markers in their blood. In fact, there is even a case on record where a healthy, active research scientist had antibody levels twice as high as the CEBV patients he was examining! Clearly, we need a more specific probe.

Scientists now believe that the best way to pin down this diagnosis is to examine not just one blood marker, but a whole family of them. When your body meets a foreign viral invader like EBV, it doesn't create just one "magic bullet" antibody to deal with the enemy. It goes through several distinct phases of antibody production, just as a field general may use different kinds of artillery at different moments in a battle. Each is tailored to attack a different part of the invader. The three stages are:

1. Antibodies to the virus's outer "envelope," called *VCA*
2. Early-stage antibodies to the virus, called *EAD* and *EAR*
3. Antibodies to the nucleus of the virus, called *EBNA*

(Don't worry, there won't be a quiz! I'm just presenting this for the scientifically inclined among you.) While the details are highly technical, if you sketched them out on a graph, they would look something like this:

## PROGRESSION OF EPSTEIN-BARR INFECTION

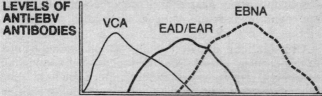

**LEVELS OF ANTI-EBV ANTIBODIES**

VCA    EAD/EAR    EBNA

**DURATION OF ILLNESS**

This means that instead of looking at a thin cross-section, we must look at a whole family portrait of the EBV-family antibodies. Measuring the relative proportions of the early- (VCA), middle- (EAD/EAR), and resolution-stage (EBNA) antibodies and comparing the various ratios and concentrations is the best way your doctor can view what is really going on—and find out whether your symptoms are indeed due to EBV.

As I am sure your doctor will agree, such sophisticated assays are best done by people with the specific technical knowledge to assess them. That usually means an immunological specialist with an expertise in viral syndromes.

It is not that your own doctor cannot do this, but knowing how to judge these laboratory values is an art as much as it is a science, and it often requires a practitioner who has seen a wide variety of these EBV blood profiles. I suggest you discuss this with your doctor.

One last note. I have talked in detail about these blood tests, but I don't want to leave you with the idea that a physician would give you a diagnosis of CEBV based solely on lab values. To make the most accurate determination, your doctor will look at your symptoms, history, and what he or she knows about how you deal with disease—all of this in addition to your blood tests. A complex diagnosis, to be sure, but CEBV is a complex disease.

## The Terrible Trio

So far I have spoken about CEBV as though it were one, absolutely distinct disease. Well, now that you have passed the beginner's course, I can admit it: That's only half the story.

Or a third, actually. Because if you look back at the title to this chapter, you can see that I mentioned a viral trio, of which CEBV is the first member. Since you have come this far (pat yourself on the back for becoming such an instant expert on this viral phantom), I now want briefly to round out the picture about what we know of this trio, where CEBV fits in, and, most important, what you can do about them.

The closer we look at CEBV, the murkier its role becomes. You remember what the scientists said at Incline Village—that they could neither prove nor disprove CEBV's role. Well, that finding is coming up more and more often. In other words, we know CEBV does something and that it is undoubtedly a main culprit in this drama. But we suspect something else is going on, as well.

That's where the viral trio comes in. It has two other members, both in the herpes family. The first is *cytomegalovirus*—or, as doctors call it, *CMV*. Like EBV, CMV is very widespread, and between 40 and 80 percent of Americans are thought to carry it. In Albany, New York, for example, 45 percent of adults have it, but in Houston, Texas, fully 79 percent do.

Experts now believe that CMV plays an integral—perhaps even the central—role in the viral syndrome we have discussed in this chapter. Late-breaking research suggests that the causes are far more complex than we had originally thought. CMV may play a role as a viral co-conspirator, working in concert with EBV to make people sick with the long-lasting, debilitating viral syndrome. Some CDC researchers even believe that EBV is not the real culprit at all, but merely a sidekick of CMV, which does the real immune damage. One of these may set the stage by lowering your immune function, thus, like a Trojan horse, opening the door to another viral invader so that it can come in and do its viral dirty work.

Right now, the clues for such viral cooperation are tantalizing. The circumstantial evidence that CMV conspires in the viral syndrome seem to grow with every new research paper. One study looked at a group of patients with severe fatigue symptoms and a blood profile showing active EBV infection. They found that almost nine out of ten of the patients *also* showed antibody evidence of active CMV infection!

Likewise, CMV has been linked to AIDS. We know that virtually 100 percent of people with AIDS secrete and transmit CMV. In the early phases of AIDS research, it was thought by some that CMV could be in some way the cause of that deadly disease. Now new research published within the last year in the *Journal of the American Medical Association* suggests that CMV and EBV may act as partners of the AIDS virus, setting the stage for demolishing your body's immune defenses.

Clearly, we do not yet understand exactly how the damage is done, but every day we identify new links in this devastating viral chain. What seems clear is that CMV keeps showing up at the scene of these contagious crimes, hanging out like some shifty viral henchman, far too often for comfort.

As far as its symptoms go, the CMV viral syndrome appears virtually identical, in every particular, to what we have seen with CEBV. The extraordinary lassitude it creates, the recurring headaches, swollen glands, and fever, its mysterious, prolonged course and stubborn tenacity—all are hallmarks that this trio of teammates appear to share equally. Whether they are different manifestations of the same underlying disease, identical counterparts, or related to some yet-unidentified third factor remains to be seen.

## Hot News from the Lab: HBLV

If there is a mysterious third player in this viral drama, it may be the newest member of this viral threesome. It is so new, in fact, that it was discovered only nine months before this book went to press! Called HBLV, for human B-cell lymphotropic virus, it is still so hot from the researchers' laboratories that we understand very little about it. It was first isolated by colleagues of the scientific team that found the HIV virus that is thought to cause AIDS. They looked at the blood cells of six people, all suffering from different immune-system disorders, and discovered a hitherto-unknown viral agent. There is not yet any commercially available diagnostic blood test, so we do not know how widespread the virus is. But preliminary findings reported by one researcher suggest that it may be present in as many as one-quarter of the population of some cities. We do not yet know, however, what role, if any, this new virus may play in the viral fatigue syndrome.

Recent investigations into the newly discovered HBLV have actually opened a door on a whole new direction for research. Dr. David Purtillo, a nationally recognized virologist, has found a link between CEBV and a new family of viruses. These are the "adenoviruses," best known as the culprit of the common sore throat. Most of us—70 percent—have these viruses, and most of the time our immune systems assure that we don't get sick and show symptoms. When they do, they usually affect the upper respiratory tract, giving us fevers and the scratchy throats of a flu.

But now it appears the common adenoviruses may conspire in some way to activate EB virus, and so cause the chronic fatigue symptoms that can be so devastating. Or it may be that they only do this in those whose immune systems are already weakened. In any case, one group of researchers is now focusing on these adenoviruses as possible culprits in the Incline Village mystery epidemic.

The more we learn about the viruses behind chronic fatigue syndrome, the more complex the picture becomes. We already have an alphabet soup of possible candidates, and it's my guess that things are likely to get more complex before we fully sort them out.

Scientists hope that as we delve further into the mysteries of these viral marauders, we will learn more about how they interrelate and cooperate. But the main point to note—and it is a source of great hope—is how astoundingly quickly research in this area is progressing. The story we started in the tiny Nevada town is now being played out in gleaming laboratories across the country. I have no doubt that by the time you will read these pages, we will know much more about the relationships of these virulent viruses.

## What Can You Do Now?

No matter how exciting the tidings from the research frontier, it is clearly news for tomorrow. It doesn't help much if you, or someone in your life, needs help *now*. In these last few pages, I want to focus on what you and your doctor can do *right now*. Believe me, if you or someone you love are one of the thousands suffering the crushing fatigue of the viral syndrome, tomorrow seems as if it will never come.

Perhaps the first step is to have the thorough medical and immunological workup necessary to establish a diagnosis of viral syndrome. Whether the culprit is one of the viral trio—EBV, CMV, or HBLV—or turns out to be another related virus, the diagnosis can help in several ways.

First, and most obvious, it tells you that no, you are not crazy. One of the foremost authorities in this field, a physician at the National Institutes of Health who has seen as many EBV patients as anyone, put it well in a recent professional journal: "Merely informing patients of an organic basis for their condition can be psychologically helpful" ("Chronic EBV Suspected in Recurring Throat Infections and Fatigue," *Medical World News*, Nov. 26, 1984, p. 71). After the despair and frustration usually experienced by viral victims, hearing this diagnosis is usually a breath of fresh air and a huge relief. It can be healing all by itself to know there is a cause, albeit a little-understood one, for your malaise.

But even more important is what you can *do* about it. Unfortunately, when it comes to a cure, there is little even the best physicians can offer. Several antiviral drugs are now being tried, with mixed results. One is acyclovir, a drug developed to attack the herpesvirus. Another prescription agent, Cimetidine (also known as Tagamet), is a commonly prescribed ulcer medication, but it may also have some effect on EVB virus. Another drug, DHPG, has been used with some success to stop CMV infections in people whose immune system had been shattered by AIDS or other diseases. (In case you want to impress friends, the official name of the drug is 1, 3-dihydroxy-2-propoxymethyl guanine. Now you see why it goes by the name DHPG!)

A recent bit of research, one that crossed my desk just as this book was going to press, may hold some hope for CEBV victims. A researcher at the Jewish Center for Immunology and Respiratory Medicine is launching a study to determine if a product called transfer factor may hold the key to ending CEBV suffering. Transfer factor is something of a medical mystery. We have known about it for more than forty years, yet still have no idea how—or even whether—it works. Distilled from the blood of someone who has fought off an infectious disease, transfer factor can be injected into another person suffering from the same disease. Somehow, it seems to help the recipient's body rally its immune defenses. Just why and how it works remains a mystery, but the hope is that by using transfer factor from people who have recovered from infectious mononucleosis (also caused by the EB virus), we may be able to help those with the chronic form of EBV. The first tests, on a group of only six patients, showed promise, so the doctors are expanding the trial to thirty patients. We should know sometime in 1988 if this transfer-factor approach holds a possible key for CEBV sufferers.

There is some hope that we can develop a vaccine, one that will slot into the receptors on your immune cells and fill them up so that the invading viruses find no way into the cells. Other vaccines would spur the body to create antibodies that can wipe out the invading viruses before it can enter your immune cells. Such a vaccine is already being developed by the British researcher Dr. Epstein, against the Epstein-Barr virus that bears his name. Early reports suggest such a vaccine may be available for use in humans sometime within the next year. If that works, it might mean that CEBV becomes an obsolete disease viral syndrome for the children of future generations.

But for now, lacking an effective drug or vaccine, what can the hapless viral victim do? I think the answer is, "Plenty." We have seen an alphabet soup of viral syndromes, caused by EBV, CMV, HBLV, or some other viruses. Yet all of them bear one thing in common. They attack the cells of your immune system. That seems to be the one common denominator of the viral fatigue syndrome. That is also the key to vanquishing it.

If all of these attack your immune system, you must do everything possible to boost it again, so that it can rally to fight off the invading viruses. That means strengthening your immune troops. There are many ways to do that, and I have written a whole book on the subject *(Dr. Berger's Immune Power Diet).*

Obviously, that topic is far too complex to cover adequately here. But I do want to outline at least briefly the basic principles of this multifaceted approach to immune building, so that you can begin to put it into effect in your own life.

First: Give yourself all the micronutrients—vitamins, minerals and amino acids—your immune cells need to work efficiently and powerfully. That means balancing doses of vitamins C, E, and A, the B complex vitamins, and such crucial immune-boosting minerals as zinc, magnesium, and iron.

Second: Avoid the toxins—dietary, chemical, and environmental—that can interfere with optimal immune action. That means avoiding heavy metals, such as lead, cadmium, and arsenic; it means making appropriate dietary changes, including the removal of trigger foods to which your immune cells react, and it means paying careful attention to an immune-balanced regime.

Third: Stop smoking. Every puff weakens your immune cells.

Fourth: Reduce undue immune stresses. Heavy psychological pressures, work stresses, too-strenuous exercise, even too much sunlight—all can tax the body's reserves or directly weaken the immune system. The better job you do of building them out of your life and replacing them with safe and sane immune habits, the less your chances of becoming a viral victim. We have come full circle, so that we now understand that such grandmother's bromides as getting enough sleep, moderate exercise, and eating a balanced diet in fact embody a profound scientific truth.

Of course, a fully balanced immune plan requires far more detail than we can go into here. (That's why it's a book in itself.) But what is important to realize is that until medical science comes up with a better answer, the best available means of controlling these viral syndromes—indeed, of strengthening yourself against all disease—is the conscious, careful rebuilding of your own immune defenses. The best news of all, of course, is that you are the one who has control over such a program. It's entirely up to you, in cooperation with your doctor.

I want to close this chapter on a personal note. We have come a long way since we began with the Nevada virus. I know, from personal experience, just how frustrating it is to meet patients whose lives have been shattered, whose energy is wasted, and who totter on the edge of despair with a condition no doctor can really help. I know what it is like to explain to a concerned family that "you have something we can't help." It is the hardest thing a doctor ever has to say, and it never gets any easier. Having seen this happen so many times, I wish more than anyone that we had the medical tools at hand to help such people.

But we do not—yet. I firmly believe that until we do, the single most promising answer is the personal, immune-boosting approach. It is the best and most effective way I know to ensure that you and yours won't fall victim to the many viral illnesses that sap energy and sour lives. It is what I have seen work, for myself, for my family, and for my patients. Don't you owe it to yourself—and those you love—to give it a try?

## For Deeper Study

Both because I know of no suitable lay books on the subject of EBV, CMV, and the viral syndrome and because our information is changing so quickly, this is a different kind of list than the recommended reading lists I have included in other chapters. The first listings are sources that can help you learn more. The second section, "For Your Doctor," includes articles that are more technical. I include these so that you can make them available to your physician, in case you feel he or she might benefit from knowing more about the research on this phantom.

## For You

"Why Are You So Tired?" *American Health,* May 1987, p. 54.

"Malaise of the 80's." *Newsweek,* October 27, 1986, p. 105.

"Viruses, the Lurking Menace." *Medical World News,* May 12, 1986.

National CEBV Association.

"CEBV—Chronic Epstein-Barr Virus Syndrome."
A basic, questions-and answers pamphlet for CEBV sufferers from the National CEBV Association, Inc., P.O. 230108, Portland, Oregon 97223.

A newsletter, *The National CEBV Reporter,* is also available and is the best lay source for current news on CEBV "Guidelines for Interpreting EBV Antibody Titers."

You can also get a complete guide to CEBV test results for you and your doctor.

## For Your Doctor

Symposium on Chronic Epstein-Barr Virus Disease. *Annals of Internal Medicine* 103 (December 1985): 951.

"Evidence for Active Epstein-Barr Virus Infection in Patients with Persistent Unexplained Illnesses: Elevated Anti-Early Antigen Antibodies." *Annals of Internal Medicine* 102 (January 1985): 1.

"Persisting Illness and Fatigue in Adults with Evidence of Epstein-Barr Virus Infection." *Annals of Internal Medicine* 102 (January 1985): 7.

"Chronic Mononucleosis: Pitfalls in Laboratory Diagnosis." *Human Pathology* 17, no. 1 (January 1986).

"A Cluster of Patients with Mononucleosis-Like Syndrome." *Journal of the American Medical Association* 257, no. 17 (May 1, 1987): 2,297.

"EB or Not EB—That Is the Question." *Journal of the American Medical Association* 257, no. 17 (May 1, 1987): 2,335.

"Sporadic Postinfectious Myasthenia." *Canadian Medical Association Journal* 133 (October 1, 1985).

"Depression Correlated with Cellular Immunity in Systemic Immunodeficient Epstein-Barr Virus Syndrome." *Journal of Clinical Psychiatry* 47, no. 3 (March 1986).

# 13

# Foods and Phantoms

In this chapter, we are now ready to make the acquaintance of the final member of the phantom family. As we will see, understanding and defeating this phantom holds the key to keeping yourself maximally healthy, vital, and functioning at your top capacity.

If you have read my other books, you know that the primary area of my medical specialization and expertise is the fascinating and little-understood field of hidden (or "occult") food sensitivities. You may have even been wondering whether I would touch on them here. Well, don't be disappointed; of course I will.

I know of no better example of a biological phantom than these hidden food sensitivity responses—unexpectedly common, often overlooked, elusive to diagnose, and despite their growing presence in the medical world of research, journals, and conferences, still very sketchily understood by many, if not most, medical practitioners. In short, food sensitivities bear all the identifying marks of a true phantom.

In my own medical practice, having seen thousands of patients over a decade, I have observed time and time again the many people who have had their lives literally turned upside-down by the insidious and destructive symptoms created by these damaging food reactions.

But more important, those years of experience have also shown me that it doesn't have to be that way, that there is a way out of this phantom's grip. And that is the real message of this chapter.

The topic of food sensitivities is an immense and complex one and, if you are like many of my patients, one that I suspect you may already know something about. I know that many of the people I see in my practice and the thousands of others I have met across the country who have read my earlier writing actually know *more* about this subject than some medical professionals do! That is not because their doctors aren't informed—not at all—but because these patients have recognized themselves in others' stories and so have made a personal commitment to becoming experts, learning enough to overcome their own phantom.

So even if some of this material sounds familiar, I suspect that you might find a refresher course helpful. If, on the other hand, you are new to it, an overview is doubly important. For that reason, the first part of this chapter provides a quick summary. Then, in the rest of the chapter, I have tried to give you a roundup, taking up where other books have left off. You can consider it a graduate course, aimed at bringing you up-to-date on the newest research and findings, bringing together the most recent theories experts now believe.

As always, if you are interested in delving more into the basics of this fascinating topic, you will find resources to do that in the "For Deeper Study" section at the end of this chapter.

So, whether this is new to you or you're just taking the graduate course, whether you are a novice or an old hand, remember that all of this is geared to one thing: helping *you* make the changes—with your doctor's help—to lay this phantom to rest once and for all *in your life*.

## Tasty . . . But Toxic?

First, let's take a quick look of what I mean by the term *food sensitivity*. You may be one of the many people who already know that you have a particularly acute reaction to certain food items, such as the man who swells up and gets nauseous when he eats cabbage or the woman who breaks out in hives after eating two strawberries. These are classic, medically recognized acute food allergies, well known to physicians, and their symptoms can take a wide variety of forms.

But many medical practitioners are now coming to the dawning realization that such responses are really only the most visible tip of a much greater iceberg of negative food sensitivities. Submerged below them lie a whole range of toxic, noxious reactions that all of us get in response to substances we eat and drink, reactions that *can be so subtle, you do not even recognize them, yet that take a significant toll on your health.*

Although it has been eighty-five years since food reactions were first scientifically demonstrated, until rather recently the medical establishment has only recognized the first, most obvious kinds of food sensitivities—those in the visible tip of the iceberg. But now they are beginning to wake up to the full extent of these problems. To wit, the final report issued last year by an expert panel of the Institute of Food Technologists came to this conclusion: "True food allergies represent only a fraction of the individual adverse reactions to foods" (Status Summary, Institute of Food Technologists' Expert Panel on Food Safety and Nutrition, "Food Allergies and Sensitivities," *Food Technology,* Sept. 1985, p. 65).

But just recognizing that these reactions exist is not enough, for there remains an awful lot we still don't understand. We do not know why sometimes, instead of unleashing the classic histamine-based response of a true allergy, these foods manage to short-circuit your body's allergy alarm altogether. We don't know exactly why or how they set off their chain reaction of biochemical disturbances and create so many chronic, serious symptoms. But I do know that these symptoms account for the great and hidden bulk of the sickness and ill health caused by the foods we eat.

We also know that these responses are highly individualized, as though Nature had tailor-made them for each one of us. That means there can be no across-the-board, blanket prescription for treating them, because you have your very own unique set of potential problem foods—everybody does. A given food that may cause tremendous medical, physiological, or psychological problems for you may not create even a ripple for your mate or your children. Yet when you ingest one of your own "trigger foods," it can unleash significant biochemical reactions with constituents of your bloodstream, especially the vital white blood cells of your immune system.

The result can be an enormous range of symptoms, affecting virtually every one of your body's biological systems. In addition to the immune system, phantom food reactions can make themselves felt in your gastrointestinal, urinary, and nervous systems; in your blood, skin, and hair; even in balances of vital neurotransmitters and hormones. They can even affect your mood, mental capacities, and psychological and emotional stability.

Considering that they can create such a wide range of problems, these sensitivities are often frustratingly hard to detect, as we will see. It is this fact that makes them the persistent, pernicious phantoms they are—and why it is so crucial that you take an active role in understanding them and knowing what you can do to end the "food-phantom" cycle.

## What's in a Name?

As with many other newly discovered phantoms, the medical establishment is a long way from having a good grasp on the problem of food sensitivities. Our understanding is so basic, in fact, that authorities can't even agree on exactly what to term this phantom! It is a telling measure of our scientific confusion that medical experts have yet even to accept a standardized terminology for the effects that so many of us see every week among our patients.

To give you an idea of how much flux this area is in, I sampled just three research papers that have crossed my desk recently. My goal was to cull out a representative list of terms now in current use describing food sensitivities in the medical and scientific press. From these papers alone, it's easy to see that this phantom has a multitude of faces:

| | |
|---|---|
| Food allergy | Secondary food sensitivity |
| Nonallergic food reaction | Food idiosyncrasy |
| Food intolerance | Food sensitivity |
| Metabolic food reaction | Anaphylactoid reaction |
| Allergylike food | Adverse food reaction |
| intoxication | Food hypersensitivity |

Confused? I expect so. And who can blame you? As to the exact differences and similarities among all these terms, nobody really agrees. Too often these terms are bandied about, often interchangeably, with little common agreement about where one stops and the other begins. I reprint this list not to make you an expert on medical nomenclature, but to emphasize the very obvious point that our best researchers are very far from having a concise, standardized way of describing this problem, let alone treating it! Definitions vary from researcher to researcher, country to country, and duplications and redundancies abound. (My own definition is simple: A food sensitivity is a response to a substance that, taken in an equal amount, is harmless to other people. That's the definition I'll be using throughout this chapter, and the most helpful one I know to give you a handle on the food phantom.)

The moral of this long list of medical names is clear. There would not be so many names if there were not some significant phenomenon occurring. No matter what we call it, we are clearly seeing a significant problem at work here. It is a medical frontier that has excited the curiosity of a wide number of researchers, clinicians, nutritionists, and doctors. For my part, while I appreciate the need for standardized labels, I am much less concerned about what we call it than about what we do about it.

## How Much, How Often?

Considering that we don't even know what to call it, it's not surprising that experts also can't agree on how common it is. In the time since I have written my other books dealing with this subject, there have been many research papers and articles. Because there are so many, I thought it would be instructive to compare what they say about the incidence of this problem. Look at just a few of the highly variable figures:

- A recent paper in the *Journal of the American Dietetic Association* puts the incidence of frank food allergies at 3 to 20 percent of babies and 3 percent of adults.
- From a Harvard Medical School researcher, a report that 1 percent of adults have allergies to cow's milk and that one in twenty newborn babies have adverse reactions to one or more foods. Of the people studied, more than half were women, and half were age twenty or younger.
- An article by a professor of pediatrics at Duke University reports that parents in the United States and Scandinavia believe that 20 percent of their children have adverse reactions to foods and that one-quarter of adult patients with asthma and hay fever had food-related allergic symptoms.
- Two-thirds of the nurses studied in one test group at the University of Michigan Medical School Allergy Clinic had "obvious" reactions to some foods.

This sampling of recent studies shows how very much we still have to understand. You can take your pick: Is the true incidence 3 percent, 20 percent, or two-thirds? The case gets clearer when you start looking not at the general population, but at people who actually complain of symptoms. Then the link to food sensitivity becomes inescapable:

- Just this month an article in the *Journal of the American Dietetic Association* found that 86 percent of a group of children with skin problems (dermatitis) tested positive for hypersensitivity to one or two foods.
- One Oklahoma researcher studying the link between allergy and mental illness examined fifty-three patients with psychiatric symptoms and found that 92 percent of them suffered psychiatric symptoms after eating certain foods. In the same article, a New York allergy specialist frankly estimates, "At least half the patients in mental hospitals have cerebral allergies. If we could only get to them and approach their disease as an allergic problem, I strongly believe we could help clean out the mental hospitals" (Nick Gonzales, "What's Eating You?" *Family Health,* Nov. 1977, p. 22).
- The former chairman of the Food Allergy Committee of the American College of Allergy, in a recent interview, said, "I am convinced that two-thirds of migraines are food related" (Sandra Blakeslee, "Studies Bolster Link of Food and Migraines," *The New York Times,* Jan. 7, 1986, p. 1).

The bottom line? These hypersensitivity responses are clearly frequent and without a doubt real. The more research that is done, the more we begin to appreciate just how widespread they are and the range of symptoms they can cause.

## How They Hide

Still, they remain phantoms for several reasons. First, the more we learn, the more we see that these reactions do not fall neatly into one simple class. Instead, they comprise several types. One research paper, published by the

Institute of Food Technologists' Expert Panel on Food Safety and Nutrition, reports two distinct kinds of food reactions: frank allergies and other, nonallergic reactions. The latter ones are then divided into six additional types! With so many distinct processes possibly going on, no wonder traditional methods of allergy testing often do not get to the bottom of people's food phantoms.

A second way these phantoms hide is that they often take their time about manifesting themselves. Unlike most allergies, which happen during or relatively soon after we are exposed to the offending substance, the onset of many food sensitivities may be delayed for hours, even days. In one article on food-caused migraines, it was reported that the headaches may not occur for *two or three* days. Obviously, this lag makes it much harder to draw cause-and-effect links between what you eat and how you feel and function. (If you don't believe me, try this: List what you ate for lunch and dinner two days ago. I'd be amazed if you had accurate recall; very few of my patients have.)

The third way this phantom can hide so successfully is that we really have no reliable and foolproof way to test for it. To be sure, there exist several kinds of tests: radioallergosorbent (RAST), cytotoxic, sublingual, skin tests, and the like. But we are now coming to understand that each method has its drawbacks and that none really works as well as it should to isolate the more subtle food sensitivities. (In fact, later in this chapter we'll look at how you and your doctor can find a testing method that you can use.)

In general, in the hands of most practitioners these food sensitivity tests are not sufficiently accurate or reliable—just one more way that these food sensitivities remain such hard-to-pin-down phantoms.

## News from the Research Frontiers

Not all the debate has centered around such academic issues as what to call these phantoms, how they are best classified, and what tests to use to diagnose them. At the same time, other researchers have been moving ahead, putting these theories to work. From laboratories across the world, they have been unearthing some very promising and exciting results:

• A psychiatrist at the University of Chicago Medical Center reported on sixty-five people, forty-five of whom were hospital patients, whose mood and behavior seemed to vary greatly after they ate certain foods. The doctor found a "significant correlation" between mood changes—including irritability, depression, and fatigue—and the ingestion of trigger foods, such as wheat and milk.

• From the University of California–Los Angeles, a psychologist reports that giving patients selected foods directly affected their emotional states, making some angry, lethargic, and depressed.

• British physicians, reporting in *The Lancet,* conducted a blind, placebo-controlled study on fifty-three patients suffering from serious, crippling rheumatoid arthritis. It showed that when the doctors removed certain trigger foods from the diets of these patients, patients reported "significant improvement" in their symptoms, including morning stiffness, joint pain, and walking mobility.

• Australian researchers studied a group of women arthritis sufferers who had had the disease for up to fifteen years. All the patients' symptoms worsened when they were "challenged" with such common trigger foods as eggs, wheat, potatoes, and beef.

• The *British Medical Journal* reports the case of a mother of three children who had suffered from progressive, crippling rheumatoid arthritis for more than a decade. Although she registered no particular allergies to dairy products on standard skin tests, her doctors asked her to abstain from eating dairy products—milk and cheese. Within three weeks, her symptoms dropped dramatically. For the first time in years, she was able to walk without pain, felt herself regaining her hand strength, and stopped taking anti-inflammatory medications. As an experiment, she reintroduced dairy products into her diet—and within twelve hours her severe symptoms returned. At the time of the study she had been living symptom-free for several months.

• Doctors in El Paso, Texas, examined a group of adults with a history of crippling migraine headaches. Fully one-third improved when they avoided trigger foods to which they were sensitive, and six were able to eliminate their headaches completely.

These and other recent studies point to one inescapable conclusion: Eliminating sensitivity-causing trigger foods has already helped many people rid themselves of serious, even debilitating symptoms—often symptoms that had haunted their lives for years. In many cases, these symptoms had shattered and warped not only their lives, but those of their mates and families. Now that the medical evidence is pouring in, the time has come to put these findings to work . . . in your own life.

## The Symptoms of Sensitivity

You may be saying that you don't have migraines or arthritis, so surely food sensitivities don't apply to you. But the fact is that those are only two of the many symptoms these sensitivities can cause. Indeed, when we look at how many and varied the reactions to food sensitivities can be, all of a sudden the true breadth and seriousness of this phantom begins to hit home. Truthfully, it is a very rare American indeed who can completely discard the possibility that this phantom may play a real—and hidden—role in his or her own life and health.

I have distilled the list below from a series of research papers, clinical findings, and case reports in the medical literature. Each has been associated, frequently or rarely, with adverse reactions to the seemingly nutritious foods we eat every day.

**Gastrointestinal:**
Nausea
Cramps
Bloated abdomen
Vomiting
Diarrhea
Constipation

**Respiratory:**
Asthma
Throat swelling
Runny nose
Shortness of breath
Wheezing
Sneezing
Coughs

**Skin:**
Swelling and puffiness
Hives
  Rash
  Eczema

**Mental/Psychological**
Anxiety
Schizophrenia
Tension
Fatigue
Behavioral disorders
Nervousness
Weakness
Sleep disturbance
Hyperactivity
Depression

**Other:**
Itchy eyes, nose
Arthritis joint pain
Muscle cramps
Menstrual irregularities
Headache
Migraine
Obesity

Although this looks like a vast laundry list of symptoms, not all of them are equally common. By far the three largest involve skin, breathing, and digestion. One study charted reactions to common foods and found that these three areas represent the great majority of food sensitivity reactions (see opposite). (The total exceeds 100 percent because many patients had several different food sensitivity reactions.)

In another study, two-thirds (64 percent) of patients with food reactions manifested asthma and skin reactions, such as eczema; an additional 22 percent suffered from other skin reactions, such as swelling and hives; and about 14

## COMMON FOOD SENSITIVITY REACTIONS

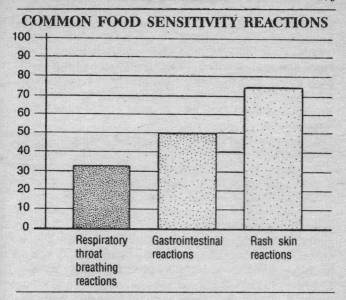

percent suffered severe gastrointestinal symptoms, including nausea, cramping, vomiting, and diarrhea.

### Oh, My Aching Head

One of the other prime areas where food sensitivities rear their ugly symptoms concerns migraine headaches. If you have never experienced one, it is hard to fully appreciate the trauma of these attacks. Often coming on without warning, these pounding headaches can bring even the strongest of people to a moaning, pain-ridden state. The searing agony can make it impossible to work, to be social, to do anything but lie in a quiet, darkened room for hours until the migraine passes.

Happily, many special clinics have sprung up around the country to help migraineurs. From many of them is coming a clear message: that certain of the foods we eat every day play a pivotal role in many migraine attacks. Fortunately, many respected physicians are coming to understand this link. Recently the former chairman of the Food Allergy Committee of the American College of Allergy reflected this growing understanding in an interview I read. He estimated the percentage of food-related migraines to be not one-third or even one-half, but fully *three-quarters* of all migraines!

This new knowledge has meant that doctors are learning to attack these debilitating migraines at their source: the dinner table. In a study reported from London, physicians treated a group of eighty-eight children with severe migraine problems. For these children, their crippling headache attacks were more than a bother. They interfered with their development at home, at school, with their classmates. Curious about the dietary connection, the researchers put the children on special diets designed to eliminate the foods to which each child was shown to be sensitive. In several months the results were in and were quite impressive: Of the original eighty-eight children, *eighty-two of them—93 percent—had no further symptoms whatsoever!* In a study in our own country, reported in the *Annals of Allergy,* Texas physicians treated forty-three long-term migraine sufferers with individually tailored, hypoallergenic diets. Again, the results were dramatic: Thirty percent of them showed a clear and marked improvement in their symptoms.

These studies and many others like them suggest that the link between migraines and food sensitivities is at last becoming clearer. More and more, it seems, the most potent weapon in our arsenal against these killer headaches is not a miracle drug, but simple, effective "dietary design" that builds migraines out of your life, once and for all.

## The Food-Mood Link

Migraines are not the only way that food sensitivities can be "all in your head." It has become evident that they also can play an important role in a variety of psychological disturbances and disorders, ranging from mania to depression. Unfortunately, all too often, the food link in such disorders is completely overlooked.

In truth, that is one of the prime reasons food sensitivities can remain the phantoms they are. Because they masquerade behind a facade of dramatic mental illness, all too often doctors never even get around to considering food sensitivities as the true cause of psychological imbalance. As with so many of the phantoms, hapless victims of food sensitivities may acquire a whole basket of psychological diagnoses, ranging from neuroses, hypochondria, and depression to full-blown psychosis, even schizophrenia.

Yet, for a certain percentage of these people, the actual root of their pain and suffering may be due to adverse reactions to items in their diet. Instead of suffering with hives, itching, or nausea, these unfortunates may manifest what are called cerebral allergies, where food sensitivities disturb the delicately balanced equilibrium of brain chemicals and neurotransmitters. For these people, the root of their mental disease may be found no farther than at the end of their fork!

Nobody knows just how frequently this happens. But one physician expert estimated over a decade ago that *one-half* of those in mental hospitals have some kind of cerebral allergies to the food they eat! What I find astounding is that, in the time since, when we have learned so much more about the interactions of food and mood, there still remains little thorough or systematic effort to test and diagnose food sensitivities among the mentally ill.

Yet at the same time, other studies suggest that a food-mood truth is definitely at work. One researcher, Dr. William Philpott, looked at fifty-three schizophrenic patients. He found that the overwhelming majority—*92 percent!*—

had a noticeable psychological reaction to one or more foods. For these psychiatric patients, the trigger foods that set them off were dismayingly common: Two-thirds of the people reacted to wheat; one-half responded to either corn or milk.

A more recent study was conducted by a psychiatrist researcher at the University of Chicago Medical Center. The trial was scrupulously designed with a double-blind mechanism, to ensure scientifically valid comparisons. Again, the doctors looked at mood changes related to foods. This time, they studied not just forty-five psychiatric patients, but twenty volunteers with no previously reported food problems. Once again, the results were tantalizing. A majority of the subjects showed what the author called "highly significant" correlations between mood changes—including irritability, depression, difficulty in concentrating, and fatigue—and common food items, such as milk and wheat.

In another study, this one from California's renowned Langley Porter Psychiatric Institute, a psychologist examined these subtle food-mood links. Early research findings suggested that his subjects experienced a clear and noticeable emotional response to challenges with specific foods. Sometimes they felt elated and "up," but subjects also reported feelings of anger, irritability, depression, and mental sluggishness.

It goes without saying that you don't need to be a psychiatric patient to feel such effects. What may be occurring to a greater extent in these patients is, in fact, the same thing that may be occurring in many of us: subtle (and not-so-subtle!) changes in our mood, mental functions, and emotions, intimately tied to what we eat.

When you look back at the wide range of symptoms—from physical to emotional to mental—that have been linked to foods, one can't help but begin to wonder if our dinner plates ought to bear a warning: "Caution: Contents May Be Hazardous to Your Health!"

## Get to Know the Food Phantoms

We have already seen that this is the Phantom, not of the Opera, but of the Kitchen. But at this point, you may be wondering what to do. After all, we all have to eat, right? You certainly can't eliminate the healthy, nutritious foods and try to subsist on hypoallergenic rations, all in the name of health!

I couldn't agree more. In fact, I think healthy eating is one of the supreme pleasures of human existence. But that's the key—"healthy" eating. So let us look together at the ways you can construct your diet to include the maximal possible health and exclude your food sensitivities.

Now, it is obvious that you can't fight a phantom without knowing what it is. That means that the first step is to identify the food sensitivities that might be at work in your life. Although that may seem a daunting prospect, given the variety in our modern American diets, research has given us some helpful places to start.

For example, over and over again, studies show a similar profile of foods that commonly trigger food sensitivity reactions. Culling from several studies, the list of "worst offenders" looks like this:

Milk
Eggs
Legumes, especially peanuts and soybeans
Wheat
Fish/shellfish
Corn

Of course, these six represent only the first rank of food offenders, the ones most commonly cited in the food sensitivity literature. To these I would add foods I have determined, over the years of my medical practice, also pose common risks for many people:

## Other Common Trigger Foods

Alcohol
Apples
Bananas
Bell peppers
Chocolate
Cocoa
Cheese
Citrus fruits
  Lemons
  Limes
  Oranges
  Tangerines
  Grapefruit

Coffee
Cottonseed oil
Eggplant
Hot dogs
Meat, especially beef
Nuts
Onions (white)
Paprika
Pizza
Potatoes
Squash
Tomatoes
Zucchini

## More Than Meets the Eye

I hope you won't be misled by these food lists into thinking that if you just eliminate these foods, you will have steered clear of the shoals of food sensitivities. That's not correct, for several reasons.

First, the foods I have listed here are just the most common ones, statistically, that I and other researchers have noticed may give people trouble. The real truth is, that food sensitivities are an equal-opportunity pest. Any food can be a problem for you *if you are one of those sensitive to it*. A recent report from an expert panel of the Institute of Food Technologists stated that adverse food reactions "have been linked to virtually every food in the American diet."

Now hold on—obviously, you can't eliminate every food. Who wants to be left eating nothing but water and gruel (nope, not even: gruel—made from grains, such as wheat and oats—wouldn't be allowed)? The truth is that nobody can really eliminate all of these foods.

Fortunately, nobody has to. Remember, the great majority of foods don't cause problems for the great majority of people. For you, that means that most of what you eat is probably perfectly fine. *The essential trick is simply to track down and eliminate only those food phantoms that are reacting with your particular biochemical makeup and causing problems for you.*

Before I explain how to do that, I want to touch briefly on one area that is commonly overlooked in the topic of food sensitivities (this *is* your graduate course, after all!).

## Watch for the Artificial Phantoms

So far, we have talked about how foods themselves may cause food sensitivity reactions. But often, these unpleasant biological reactions are caused not by the food themselves, but by a "little something extra" that has been added to the basic food.

In this age of hyperprocessed, ultrarefined foods, it is an open secret that an extraordinary amount of tampering has been done with your food long before you get it. The same groceries that, two generations ago, were fresh from the farm have now been preserved, colored, emulsified, stabilized, flavored, reprocessed, bleached, sterilized, and even irradiated before they get to us. Not surprisingly, we are now coming to appreciate just how much many of those processes and additives can also unleash legions of food-reaction phantoms. There is no better way of making this point than to let you peek over my shoulder at a recent review paper, published by Dr. Tak Lee, a researcher from the Harvard Medical School. In the article, Dr. Lee lists a whole rogue's gallery of food additives and contaminants: "Molds are prominent in fermented food products, and antibiotics used to treat cattle have contaminated milk. Dyes and additives . . . may cause . . . hypersensitivity reactions. . . . Preservatives [in] salads, shrimp, wine, baked goods (especially pizza and tortilla shells), and vegetable and fruit juices, may induce symptoms suggestive of allergic disease."

The more we become aware of these reactions, the more compelling grows the medical evidence:

- Studies over the last two decades have shown that the common food colorant tartrazine, otherwise known as yellow dye number 5, has been linked to hives, asthma, and swelling reactions. Although study results varied, the reactions have occurred in as few as 8 percent, and as many as 100 percent, of people studied.
- Other dyes and the flavor enhancer monosodium glutamate have been linked to severe facial swelling and a skin disfiguration known as oro-facial granulomatosis, an abnormal growth of the upper lip and cheek. In one reported case, a diet avoiding these additives helped reverse the symptoms in six months.
- Between one-half and one million Americans are sensitive to sulfites used to preserve foods. These chemicals may be listed on a food label hidden in such compounds as sulfur dioxide or sodium bisulfite; in some fast foods they may not be listed at all. But for susceptible individuals, ingesting such chemicals can create symptoms ranging from headaches and runny nose to severe gastrointestinal upset, explosive diarrhea, and potentially fatal breathing problems. More than twelve hundred cases have now been reported due to these additives, and a dozen deaths have been attributed to them. Unfortunately, sulfites have become fairly ubiquitous hitchhikers in the processed foods we eat. Among the varied sources of these sulfites: salad bars, dried fruit, shrimp, processed and dried soups, dried mixes, guacamole dip, corn syrup, wine, fruit juices, soft drinks, hominy, dried nuts, freeze-processed potatoes. If you believe that sulfites may be a problem for you, you can now get sulfite test strips, which you can carry with you.
- The "Chinese restaurant syndrome" was recognized several years ago, due to the high levels of monosodium glutamate (MSG) used in certain Oriental preparations. The symptoms can range from a mild, warm feeling

across your chest, to weakness and stiffness in your arms and legs, to upset stomach and headaches.

When it comes to additives, the research on this topic is both broad and convincing. But the important thing for you to remember is that not all additives are created equal, and some of them may have decidedly deleterious effects on your health. If you are interested in exploring this subject further, I urge you to consult the resources in the "For Deeper Study" section at the end of this chapter.

## Vanquishing Your Food Phantoms

Up until now, we have talked mostly about the food-phantom problem: what foods may cause sensitivities, what symptoms they create, how additives aggravate the problem. But now it is high time to stop talking about the problem and start talking instead about a solution—*your* solution, so that you can make sure that this food phantom no longer wreaks havoc in your life.

Perhaps what you have read so far makes you think you could be at risk for, or suffering from, food sensitivities. If that's so, the very first step is to find out if that is, indeed, true. But while that sounds sensible, it is unfortunately somewhat more easily said than done. For, as you might expect, in this cutting-edge area, the state of the art in food sensitivity testing leaves much to be desired.

Without going into all the nitpicking scientific details (which will have changed by the time this book gets to press, in any case!), the bottom line is that if you get to your doctor, you will find yourself confronted with a whole smorgasbord of kinds of tests. I have before me a whole stack of erudite and technical papers, each arguing for one type of test or another—skin tests, sublingual (under the tongue) tests, RAST blood tests, antibody tests, cytotoxic tests, hospital-isolation tests.

The problem is that no one test can do the trick, and each has some fairly significant failing. Antibody tests are not standardized; RAST and skin tests may miss up to one-half of food sensitivities; cytotoxic tests show poor repeatability; sublingual tests are too uncontrolled. One overview article, published in a recent issue of the *Journal of the American Dietetic Association*, cites six studies showing that these various means of testing don't really work. In the researchers' words, "Recent double-blind placebo-controlled studies have demonstrated the general unreliability . . . of allergy skin tests, radioallergosorbent tests, and various other methods in accurately predicting the presence of food hypersensitivity." The whole area is confusing, but the table that follows summarizes much of the current thinking.

| Type of Test | Advantages | Disadvantages |
|---|---|---|
| Isolation test (hospital inpatient) | • Best in severe cases<br>• Highly accurate<br>• Most specific | • Very expensive<br>• Requires hospital stay<br>• Disruptive to routine<br>• Takes several weeks |
| Sublingual test (under the tongue) | • Symptom-specific<br>• Reactions clear | • Time-consuming<br>• May miss some hidden food sensitivities |
| Cytotoxic (blood sample) | • Rapid results<br>• No unnecessary patient reactions<br>• Sensitive to subtle reactions | • Not highly reproducible<br>• Unsure validity |
| IgG RAST (radioimmuno-assay) | • Highly sensitive<br>• Very repro-ducible<br>• Measures anti-body reaction | • Very specialized<br>• Expensive<br>• Requires sophisticated laboratory |

| Type of Test | Advantages | Disadvantages |
| --- | --- | --- |
| Scratch- or prick-type skin tests (back or arm) | • Easily available<br>• Standardized interpretation | • Long, time-consuming<br>• Expensive<br>• Inaccurate, may miss hidden sensitivities<br>• Reactions can block each other |

As you can see, the debate rages on and on. While that may be of great interest if you are an academic doctor, I am interested in a much more immediate, and more personal, answer. For me, and for you, the real question is what about the poor person, possibly suffering from a range of severe symptoms, who is caught in the middle and needs help *now?*

Fortunately, that is a question with a happy answer. The truth is that even if you went to a physician specializing in these hidden food phantoms, one who had all of these tests at his or her disposal, that would provide only one part of the answer. Even in the best of situations, the medical tests above can really give only a partial answer to uncovering food phantoms, a rough and ready guide for your doctor.

But the remaining pieces of the puzzle—the really crucial ones—don't come from any lab or chemistry test at all. They come from you. By far the best way to see if you are a food-phantom victim, the authorities agree, is to use these tests as only part of a more in-depth workup. And the single most valuable and necessary part of that workup has nothing to do with the lab tests at all, but everything to do with you.

*The facts you can reveal about what you eat, when you have symptoms, what they are, your overall eating patterns, allergic and family history, and overall health are far more useful for tracking down and exorcising these phantoms than any single lab test.*

What does all this mean for you? Simple. It means that, for this phantom, as for so many of the others we have seen, *you* truly hold the key to your health. Working together with your doctor, you can have the key role in pinpointing which foods do what to you and consequently which to avoid.

The most advanced physicians working with food sensitivities now recommend a broad-based, holistic approach. You can expect that it will include several aspects:

- Writing down a detailed medical and allergic history
- Exploring what you note about your food reaction symptoms
- Keeping a detailed "diet diary" to track your food intake and responses (as I explained in *How to Be Your Own Nutritionist*)
- Removing potential trigger foods from your diet
- Charting any change in symptoms
- Reintroducing (or "challenging") with trigger foods to see if your symptoms recur

In short, the most powerful tools for helping to eliminate this phantom are not wonder drugs, but data and information, which you provide. You may look at this list and say, "But I could do that. Why do I need a doctor?" My answer is, of course you can do it—*absolutely*—but most of us don't.

There is no reason you can't track down these phantoms on your own, or at least get a good start at figuring out which of them may be haunting you. But the value of having a trusted doctor by your side is that he or she will help order and streamline the process, by knowing where to look, focusing on clues you may otherwise overlook, and providing an objective, informed partner in your food-phantom search.

## Treatment: Just Say No

Now comes the easy part. As with so many phantoms, once you have unmasked your food phantoms, the actual treatment for them is relatively easy. By far the great majority of experts agree that the best way to deal with food sensitivities is not through drugs or medication regimens, but by the simplest tactic of all: avoidance.

Simply knowing what you react to makes it easy to build these food items out of your diet. As you do, you can expect to see your aggravating symptoms melt away. I find that the great majority of my patients are able to maintain themselves on a stable, allergen-free diet with little problem.

If you are interested in more details about the maintenance process, I refer you to my book *How to Be Your Own Nutritionist,* which goes into the subject in some detail. But in addition to that, there are two important caveats I hope you will keep in mind:

First, watch for hidden phantoms. Often, particularly in prepared foods and restaurants, it is easy to get an unintentional dose of one of your trigger foods. And in our nation's overprocessed diet, food items can turn up hidden in all manner of seemingly unrelated foods: wheat products in salad dressings, say, or soy extracts in cookies. For that reason, it is especially important to get into the habit of reading labels scrupulously. Research shows that people who learn this skill and apply it consistently have far better luck at removing food phantoms from their lives and end up suffering far fewer bouts of sensitivity symptoms.

Second, it is important to understand that just because you react strongly to a trigger food today, it doesn't mean you will have to avoid it for the rest of your life. It appears that we develop sensitivity reactions to those foods we eat most often, as our body's way of adapting to what is essentially a dietary overdose. That means that if you lay off a trigger food for some time—often six or nine months— you give your body time to readjust. Then, after your "cold-turkey" period, you may be able to reintroduce the food, eating it in moderation. That may mean that instead of eating it every day, you consume it once every four days or so. Under such an intermittent schedule, most of my patients find they can tolerate the food substance with no ill effects.

Congratulations! Not only have you completed your graduate course in the area of food sensitivities, but you can be confident that you have an up-to-date, state-of-the-art understanding of many of the newest findings on this fascinating topic.

But, far more important, I hope you have gained information that will help you identify and defeat your own dietary phantoms. If so, and if you truly put these findings to work, I guarantee that you will feel, act, and look better than you have for years. I wish you all the best of luck in your campaign to put your food phantoms exactly where they belong—far out of your life, now and forever.

## For Deeper Study

Stuart Berger, M.D. *Dr. Berger's Immune Power Diet.* New York: New American Library, 1985.

——— . *How to Be Your Own Nutritionist.* New York: William Morrow and Company, 1986.

For more information on food additives, contact the Center for Science in the Public Interest, 1501 Sixteenth Street N.W., Washington, D.C. 20036.

# 14

# The Miracles of Mental Medicine

So far, we have concentrated mostly on the wide range of possible phantom illnesses. Now I want to broaden our focus beyond just these phantoms to look at what I consider the most promising, exciting, and tantalizing of recent medical developments. In this final chapter, we will open the door on a whole new medical frontier, one that can greatly affect both how you stay healthy and how you fight off sickness.

Imagine, some day in the not-too-distant future, that your doctor finds an unidentified mass in your abdomen. Instead of rushing you into surgery, you are given another program. First, you are ushered into a low-lit, comfortable room, where you sink into a fabulously comfortable armchair. At your side, an imaging specialist guides you through a trancelike meditation aimed at reducing the tumor inside you. Then, before you, a wall-sized video screen lights up, with a soothing program that helps you further picture your own body fighting off the tumor. In your ears, a rich soundtrack plays, tailored specifically to suggest powerful ways your body can become stronger and defeat this tumor.

After several weeks of this, your doctors add a series of thoroughly delightful, uproarious comedies, which leave you laughing until your sides ache. Every day, too, you sit with close friends and loved ones in a joint meditation aimed at making you feel loved and cherished and at healing your tumor. At the end of several weeks, the doctors can find no more trace of the original mass, and you feel entirely rejuvenated. You feel almost reborn, with a renewed sense of love and hope for your life. You have been spared death-defying operations, deadly X-radiation treatments, and disfiguring, toxic drugs. It may sound strange to us today, but every one of the above treatments has been attempted and has met with some degree of success. They are the fledgling tools of a brand-new scientific discipline, called *psychoneuroimmunology*.

In order to understand the meaning behind that long, Latinate label, a bit of history is in order. In the seventeenth century, the French mathematician René Descartes proposed a system of philosophy dividing the human organism into mind, on the one hand, and body, on the other. For four centuries, the medical establishment has accepted that dualism largely unchallenged.

But now, in the closing years of the twentieth century, as our understanding of medicine has grown more complex than ever before, we have discovered that things are not nearly so neatly compartmentalized. We are discovering a whole range of connections linking our physical and psychological selves. Like so many unused, hidden passageways, they thread between the parts of the body and mind in ways we have never suspected. Exploring these mysterious and powerful passageways is the task of psychoneuroimmunology.

The word itself breaks down into three parts: *psycho*, meaning "mind"; *neuro*, suggesting the brain and nervous system; and *immunology*, the science of how your body fights infection and cancer. Put them together and you get a tantalizing new formula for the ways we can literally "think ourselves to health." Behind its tongue-twisting label lies a simple, yet profound vision: that you can harness the untold powers of your mind as a tool for making your body well—and keeping it that way.

To be sure, the best doctors have always known this. But they didn't always have such a fancy name for it. The famed nineteenth-century physician Sir William Osler, revered as the father of modern American medicine, and the first professor of medicine at the Johns Hopkins Medical School, put it in these world:

> Faith in drugs and methods is the great stock in trade of the profession. . . . While we doctors often overlook or are ignorant of our own faith cures, we are just a wee bit too sensitive about those performed outside our ranks. Faith in the gods or saints cures one, faith in little pills another, hypnotic suggestion a third, faith in a plain common doctor a fourth. The faith with which we work . . . is the most precious commodity, without which we should be very badly off.

What Osler termed ''faith'' we now know to involve a complex, little-understood, and altogether fascinating network including several glands hidden deep within the brain, chemical messengers and hormones, more than a trillion immune cells, and an array of biochemical reactions so complex we are only beginning to understand them. Together, they make up the pathways of what I term *mental medicine*.

Perhaps the most intriguing question about mental medicine is, What has taken Western medicine so long to catch on? After all, there have been fascinating clues available for a very long time. From the work of native faith healers and ancient Chinese acupuncture practitioners to the medical miracles of Lourdes and the seemingly impossible physical feats of Indian yogis, it's clear that the boundaries between body and mind are not so rigid as we in the West have believed. Mental medicine may simply be a matter of learning to do what those traditional medical practitioners have long demonstrated.

In fact, we don't even have to look into exotic realms at all, for there has been plenty of tantalizing evidence about the body-mind link within our own medical tradition. From Harvard Medical School, a study reports the result of a fascinating series of tests. Heart surgeons from several institutions treated patients complaining of the pain, weakness, and heart problems of classic angina. Some of the patients underwent a standard surgical procedure in which an internal chest artery was sutured to relieve the burden on the heart. In the others, however, the surgeons only *appeared* to perform the actual operation. They gave anesthesia, made an incision in the persons's chest, but then stitched it up without actually doing anything. The surgeons' hope was to achieve the same curative results but spare the patient a serious operation—by harnessing the power of mental medicine. Then, if it didn't work, they could always do the real procedure later. Afterward the patients' health was rated, both by the patients themselves and by independent physicians.

Astoundingly, there was virtually no difference in the results! All the patients showed a 60 to 90 percent reduction in pain, enhanced quality of life, and even improved function on a standard electrocardiogram. In the words of the authors, the ratings showed conclusively that the real surgery produced "no greater benefit than the sham operation!" Other researchers repeated the test with eighteen other patients. Again, neither doctor nor patient knew which operation had been done. Yet *all* of the patients with the sham operation "emphatically described marked improvement."

For two thousand years, since the age of Hippocrates in Greece, medical science has relied on the effects of placebo medications—pills and potions that are chemically inert, yet somehow achieve remarkable cures. Scientists estimate that, across the board, placebo medications are 30 to 60 percent as effective as the medication they replace. Of course, what that really means is that placebos allow us to mobilize our body's capacity for self-healing—which is really what accounts for the impressive effectiveness of these ersatz medications.

Perhaps the most widely used tool of mental medicine is hypnosis. It has long been shown to work effectively to lower blood pressure, to relieve pain, and as a surgical anesthetic. Scientists have also found that under hypnosis, people can vary the chemical composition of their bodily fluids, including blood and liver secretions. Controlled studies have even shown hypnosis effective in nine out of ten cases in relieving skin warts that had resisted other treatments.

Sometimes, the effects of mental medicine are even more dramatic. For example, one paper, written by two distinguished surgeons, enumerates some 176 examples of complete remissions from diagnosed cancer. These doctors raise the question if these miracle cures may not be due to some interactions of the person's psyche and physical body.

We do not know why these happen, but such cases are well known to every practicing physician. From the cancer specialist who sees an inoperable tumor disappear to the family doctor whose dying patient suddenly rallies, all of us who have witnessed these mysteries cannot help but wonder what hidden force is at work. It seems likely that such resilient people are tapping into a powerful healing force that we do not yet understand—one very probably in the province of mental medicine.

## The Mind-Immune Link

As we look more closely at these instances of mental medicine, it becomes clear that one of the key ways our ideas, thoughts, and emotions affect our physical well-being is through our immune system. In fact, we are now learning that this system is vastly more sensitive to our moods and emotions than we had ever before realized.

Some of the most clear-cut evidence for the mind-immune link comes from studies on laboratory animals. One of the most typical was a study conducted some years ago at the University of California–Los Angeles. Researchers found that mice subjected to a wide variety of psychological stresses became significantly more susceptible to a wide range of infectious viruses, including herpesvirus, than mice with no stress. The message seemed clear: Psychic stress easily translates into ill health—and the immune system is the link. (Not surprisingly, the effects of such psychological stress show up throughout the body. One study even found that rats under stress have a higher incidence of cavities than their rodent companions not under stress.)

An interesting next step was taken by scientists at the Rochester Medical Center, in an experiment that showed very dramatically just how close the link is between the immune system and the mind. In this landmark study, rats were fed a distinctively flavored water along with a drug that drastically suppressed their immune system. After their immune systems had returned to normal, they were given a taste of the same flavored water, but this time without the immune-lowering drug. Amazingly, the animals' blood profiles reacted exactly the same, the number of immune antibody cells dropping steeply. The animals had actually *learned* to associate a given taste with a lowered immune system; tasting it, they went right ahead and automatically suppressed their own immune system by themselves. This dramatic study was later replicated by scientists from Harvard University Medical School.

Next, the same researchers performed an even more interesting experiment. They took a group of mice with a genetic predisposition to develop a disease called murine systemic lupus erythematosus. Like lupus in humans, the disease involves not a suppressed immune system but an overactive one. For sufferers of this disease, whether rodent or human, the treatment is to actually *reduce* the activity of the immune system, in order to bring it back into balance.

Again, the researchers used flavored water and an immune-suppressing drug to train the mice to reduce their own immune response. But this time it helped the mice. Remarkably, the trained animals were able to suppress their immune system, with the result that they actually lived significantly longer and showed fewer symptoms of their inherited condition than a control group of mice who got the same drugs but without the conditioning. Behind the complexities of the study, the result was clear and profound: Mice can actually learn to control their immune system to live longer!

## Of Mice and Men

What works for mice seems to work for human beings as well. There is an impressive and increasing body of research showing just how tightly bound our immune system is to our psychological well-being. Even more compelling, these data come not from the confines of the laboratory but from real-life situations in the real world:

- Several researchers, from England, Australia, and New York's Mount Sinai Hospital, have shown that people whose spouses have recently died have a severe, and damaging, drop in their immune system strength, as measured by their response to a standard immune-challenge test. The drop is most noticeable at one month to five months following the spouse's death.
- In a very persuasive proof of the effect stress can have on our immune system, doctors at Boston Children's Hospital examined the patterns of disease in sixteen families attending a local clinic. They found that children living in high-stress families are *more than twice as likely* to contract respiratory infections than children in low-stress families.

## Stressed-Out Students

When academic researchers want to look at the effects of stress on our immune health, they have a ready-made group from which to draw a sample: students. Not only are they available, but students also usually have periodic, regular cycles of stress and relaxation. They offer a living laboratory into the ways that psychic stress takes a toll on the body's capacity to stay well. What the students have taught their teachers is rather impressive:

- A simple study of dental students measured the levels of a particular immune-system antibody in their saliva—a key part of the body's first-line defense against cold and flu germs. They found the antibodies were significantly depleted during each exam period—the highest stress period of the students' academic year.
- Physicians in Britain sampled a group of first-year student nurses and found that those who scored highest on a psychological scale indicating unhappiness also showed a higher-than-average rate of recurrence of general illness, and specifically of herpes infections, over the course of a year.
- Doctors at West Point studied a class of fourteen hundred cadets and found they could predict which ones would come down with infectious mononucleosis based on psychological measures, including their academic performance, their motivation to perform, and whether the cadet's father was an "overachiever." It appeared that exactly those students under the greatest amount of internally generated psychological stress were the ones most likely to actually fall ill with the disease.
- In a Harvard Medical School study, physicians studied 114 undergraduate students who were under intense academic stress. The subjects divided into two clear-cut groups: "good copers," who dealt well with stress, reporting little or no psychological distress; and "poor copers," who reacted to stress with high levels of complaints, symptoms, and psychological manifestations. But the most significant difference was found in the students' blood. Tests showed that the good copers had much more powerful immune systems, and more natural killer immune cells, than the poor copers. A second study by the same research team with another group confirmed the findings. Again, it appeared that the subject's psychological coping mechanisms were directly reflected in their immune systems.

## When Your Body Attacks Itself

One suggestive proof of the mind-immune link comes from the so-called autoimmune diseases. These conditions, often life-threatening, happen when your body's natural immune-regulating mechanisms go haywire, and your body actually begins to mount an immune attack against itself. Rheumatoid arthritis is a classic example of this kind of autoimmune disease. It occurs when your body's immune cells attack your own joints, often in the knee, arms, hand, and fingers. In this crippling and disfiguring disease, the mind-immune link is particularly strong. Scientists reporting in the *British Medical Journal* studied a group of women suffering from chronic, severe rheumatoid arthritis. They found that almost 70 percent of them had experienced a traumatic emotional life event (divorce, lost job, death in family, marital problems, and so on) in the year before they developed arthritis. That rate was more than twice as high as a group of matched controls who did not report arthritis. Even more suggestive, three-quarters of the arthritis patients started having symptoms just three months after their emotional trauma.

Another similar study showed that "worry, work pressure, marital disharmony, and . . . loss of relatives could be documented immediately prior to onset of disease in nearly half the cases" of rheumatoid arthritis they examined. Some researchers have even gone so far as to describe a frequent rheumatoid arthritis personality: Someone who is dependent, who feels inadequate, with significantly blocked emotional outlets to other people. (George Freeman Solomon, "Emotional and Personality Factors in Onset and Course of Autoimmune Disease," *Psychoneuroimmunology*, [San Diego: Academic Press, 1981], p. 159).

Because rheumatoid arthritis is typical of autoimmune diseases, it is particularly provocative that it flares up so often in people with a certain psychic profile. It does not take much imagination to see that this suggests a close link between what is going on in these people's heads and what happens in their bloodstream.

The medical literature is now beginning to reflect a number of autoimmune diseases where personality factors clearly play a role. Among them, it has been suggested, are diabetes, ulcerative colitis, lupus, rheumatoid arthritis, and multiple sclerosis. In each case, researchers are now proposing, it may be that the failure of our psychological defenses, and the attendant weakening of our immune systems, may predispose us to these diseases.

## Mind Power: A New Weapon Against Cancer?

But of all the diseases involving the immune system, none is more frightening than cancer. Recent research in psychoneuroimmunology is showing just how large a role our mental set can play in keeping us safe from this dreaded, deadly disease.

A research psychologist at the University of California at San Francisco examined the link between disease and emotions among a group of people with malignant melanoma, a fatal form of skin cancer. Her study, reported in conjunction with the American Cancer Society, took patients with approximately equal chances for survival, based on standard medical tests, and gave them a battery of psychological tests. Two years later, when she looked at which patients had died, she found that they had *twice* the levels of negative emotions, such as anger, frustration, depression, dejection, anxiety, and general psychic distress, than did the patients who survived.

A continent and an ocean away, physicians in London studied sixty-nine women diagnosed with early-stage breast cancer. They divided the women into two groups: the women who faced their disease by denying it or taking a "fighting spirit" toward their illness versus those whose attitude was judged by the psychiatrists as stoic, helpless, or hopeless. Ten years later the evidence was overwhelming. Fifty-five percent of the "fighters" were still alive, as opposed to only 22 percent of the women who had stoically accepted their fate. It appears that their attitude was the factor that made it more than twice as likely for them to survive.

In our own country, a professor of psychiatry at the University of Pittsburgh School of Medicine followed a group of women with breast cancer. After seven years, she compared those who survived with those who died. She found that one of the most statistically significant differences between them was a mental one: Survivors had scored higher on a psychological test in a category called joy. One cannot help surmise that their life-loving attitude gave them the physical ability to fight back their malignancies—and win. Another team of researchers has developed a psychological test to be given to people diagnosed with malignant melanoma. Simply by using the test to gauge patients' psychological adaptation to the disease and how they coped with it, the researchers could accurately predict, in three out of four cases, whether the person would be alive one year after diagnosis!

As a physician making my living treating patients every day, I have seen for myself how powerful these forces can be. Every doctor has witnessed, as I have, the seemingly vigorous patients who, when diagnosed with a serious disease, appear simply to close off their inner strength and, like a flower past its bloom, rapidly wither and die.

What I find even more intriguing, however, are the inspiring individuals who come to me with serious, even far-advanced disease, whose prognosis is, by every medical standard, grim, yet who astound us by living out their full lives, reporting minimal pain and symptoms. Many of them have complete remissions and live for many years.

Doreen G. was one of those. When she consulted me, it was obvious that she was in intense pain, the victim of a progressive arthritic condition. The agony had become so constant that she had reluctantly taken early retirement from her job as a physical-education coach. Now even minor movements brought stabbing, excruciating pain. Every expert and textbook predicted her disease would be progressive—everybody but Doreen. I was quite struck, even on that first visit, with this woman's sheer guts to vanquish her disease.

Although I prescribed a nutritional program to help reduce her symptoms, I did not promise any great progress, so incapacitating was her pain. But I told myself that any scant relief I could offer her would be worth it.

In truth, I underestimated Doreen. Today, a year and a half later, she is again active, volunteering as a coach, working part-time, "with just an occasional twinge." Doreen gives most of the credit to the diet prescribed, but I know that's not the whole story. Doreen's sterling progress is due as much to her upbeat attitude as to any purely medical change. She is a lesson I have not forgotten. For although everything, in my medical judgment, predicted one course for her illness, I hadn't taken into account her own substantial mental reserves. When my colleagues and I discuss this case in conferences, I remember that it was Doreen, not me, who deserves credit for such a spectacular recovery.

## Mental Medicine: A New Crystal Ball?

Just as it is becoming increasingly clear that our attitudes affect the course of our disease if we do get sick, there is increasingly good evidence to suggest that your psychological makeup—your experiences, thoughts, and feelings—may even affect your chances of ever getting sick in the first place. Much of this work has been done with cancer. Researchers are now using their knowledge of mind-body links to be able to predict who will develop malignant disease and who won't—with some success.

Two psychiatrists at the University of Rochester selected a group of seemingly healthy women whose Pap smears indicated they might be at some elevated risk for developing cancer. They rated the women on one variable: whether they had "hopelessness-prone" personalities or had recently experienced intense feelings of hopelessness. Using this criterion, the doctors found that they could accurately predict, in three cases out of four, whether the women would be found to have a confirmed diagnosis of cervical cancer.

Another study looked at 110 men with undiagnosed lung complaints. By interviewing the men about their childhood, marriage, job, future plans, and recent life events, the researchers were able to predict—an average of seven times out of ten—which men would actually be diagnosed with cancer! Similar results were found by psychiatric researchers at Yale University. They followed more than 2,000 men for a period of seventeen years and found that men who were classified as depressed at the beginning of the study (based on psychological tests) were twice as likely to die from some form of cancer during the seventeen years of the study than men who were not depressed. In their abstract, they concluded, "Depression is related to the . . . mechanisms for preventing the establishment and spread of malignant cells." In other words, what makes you depressed may also raise your risk for cancer.

A similar finding is borne out by other research published in the journal *Psychosomatic Medicine*. There, researchers studied 232 patients and found a "highly significant correlation" between the magnitude of disruptive events in their lives and the onset and severity of more than forty acute illnesses, including cancer, heart attacks, strokes, diabetes, and hepatitis. By charting major life changes occurring in people's lives, they found that more than a third of the changes happened in the six months immediately before the people fell ill.

Finally, a National Institute of Mental Health study found that severe illness is commonly preceded by a period of psychological disturbance—in which people experience a feeling of giving up, hopelessness, lack of pleasure in friends and activities, a poor self-image, and a lack of "connectedness" between past, present, and future. The author terms it the Giving Up–Given Up complex.

But not all of the factors that affect our immune system operate over a few months. Some may take a whole lifetime. Several studies suggest that the presence of cancer and other immune diseases as adults may even have some relation to our experiences as a child. When British scientists tested a group of twenty-two women suffering from chronic, severe rheumatoid arthritis, they found that more than half of the rheumatoid sufferers reported significantly bad relationships with their mothers during childhood, more than twice as many as in the control group without the disease.

It may sound improbable that the psychic hurts we endure as children manifest themselves decades later as disease—yet several other fascinating studies suggest this possibility. One of them, published in the research review *Psychosomatic Medicine,* followed a selected group of male medical students after graduation and throughout their lives. It turned out that the men who went on to develop cancer later in their lives had a very specific trait in common: They reported very different family attitudes in their childhood years than did their cancer-free classmates. Universally, they showed a distinct lack of closeness with one or both of their parents. But the emotions-cancer tie is broader than just our attachment to our parents. It has been suggested by one researcher that females with breast cancer are more likely to have lost a sibling in their childhood than are other, cancer-free women.

## 'Tis Better to Have Loved . . . Or Not?

Obviously, if our relationships in childhood have such a serious effect, our relationships as adults must have an effect on our immune health as well. Indeed, according to research at the Institute of Applied Biology in New York, that may be very true. The psychologists knew that when a spouse dies, the damage makes itself felt in the immune system. Accordingly, the researchers ranked people in order of risk, starting with widowers—who, by definition, had suffered the most traumatic experience with loss. Next came divorced people, on the assumption that they had experienced an important loss, but that a "lower precentage made their marriage a major focus" (and, one assumes, because at least half of the divorced people actually may have *chosen* the separation). Married people were ranked third lowest, and single people at the bottom of the list, assuming they were least likely to have suffered the loss of an intense emotional bond of long duration. Then they compared mortality rates for cancer in women, including cancer of the breast, uterus, ovary, vagina, and other sites. Astoundingly, *the results were directly proportional to their predictions.* It may turn out that, when it comes to cancer risk at least, it is *not* better to have loved and lost than never to have loved at all!

Family relationships, depression, loss of a job, life-style changes—it seems that the list of life occurrences that can affect our health is long, if not endless. But when you think about it, all of them share a common, very deep-seated thread: our emotions. *It is how we feel about what happens to us,* our sense of loss, grief, or personal threat, that seems to be the common element in determining how and whether we will get sick—or recover.

## On the Trail of the Missing Mind-Immune Link

As we have seen in the preceding pages, the evidence for a clear-cut connection between the mind and our health is rather absolute and overwhelming. Now medical scientists want to know how, exactly, they interconnect. What is the missing link, the line between psyche and cell, that turns our ideas and feelings into the biochemical realities that direct our health, keeping us safe from cancer or heart attack? These are crucial questions, because only by knowing their answers can we begin to fine-tune the process and start using the tools of mental medicine with power and precision.

To explain the links between mind and immune system fully would require a thick medical book, a graduate course in biochemistry, and a lot more space than we have here. Furthermore, much of what I write now will be out of date by the time this book goes to press, so rapidly is this field advancing.

But I do want to give you at least a quick passing view of the very exciting components we understand so far—an incomplete picture, to be sure, but a fascinating one. Recall that the science of these interconnections is called psychoneuroimmunology—*psycho* for "mind," *neuro* for "nervous system," and *immunology* for "the immune system." Leading medical minds are now discovering the complex ways these three parts of you interact to keep you healthy . . . or sick.

It now appears that the trillion cells of your immune system, as well as the glands and organs that help create them, actually work in close concert with your nervous system. We know that the brain—the seat of the central nervous system—secretes at least four hundred complex chemical substances. They include neurotransmitters, hormones, and opiatelike substances, to name a few. They work like molecular messengers, carrying information and causing reactions within the brain. Chemically, they are compounds called neuropeptides, or peptides for short.

We learned some time ago that these same peptide messengers don't just stop at the brain. They travel through your entire body, carrying their chemical messages to organs and glands, including your thyroid, liver, spleen, heart, kidneys, digestive tract, and sex organs. What we are now learning is that *these same chemical messengers activate, instruct, and regulate our immune system as well.*

Recent discoveries are beginning to fill in many missing pieces of the mind-body puzzle:

- It has been found that some of your immune cells are sensitive to certain of your neurotransmitters. When they meet them in the blood, they "turn on" and are triggered to produce substances such as interferon, or its cousin, interleukin-2, which boosts certain functions of the immune system. To name just one, it is now known that one brain chemical, vasopressin, affects gamma-interferon production.
- Other peptides, which in the brain affect your mood and pain perception, work to attract the immune scavenger cells, called *macrophages,* to damaged tissue—such as cancer cells.
- Biochemical messengers from areas deep within your brain—the hypothalamus and pituitary glands—also work to stimulate your thymus gland to produce more of a certain kind of immune fighting cell, your T-cells.
- Prolactin, another brain chemical, helps regulate the branch of your immune system responsible for antibodies, the B-cells.

We know that there are a whole range of substances, including growth hormones, corticosteroids, and sex hormones, secreted by parts of the brain, that can be received—and presumably acted upon—by various soldiers in your body's immune forces.

Thanks to these chemical messengers, your immune cells and nervous system are constantly trading information and commands—"make more of this," "send these kinds of cells over there," "produce more of that chemical." Back and forth the messages go, carried by the faithful peptide neurotransmitter molecules. We once believed that the messages flowed all one way—from the brain to the immune system. But now we know that your immune cells themselves actually make these same peptide molecules in order to send their own messages back to the central nervous system. The cells of both immune and nervous systems receive and transmit information, using these chemical messengers.

When you consider that these same chemicals are known to play a role in mood and emotion and are even the same ones that regulate happiness, sex drive, mental functioning, sleep, depression, aggression, and all of our other brain functions—voilà—you begin to see the missing link! The closer we look, the less it seems strange that our immune system is sensitive to some conscious, and emotional, control.

It makes sense that when we have negative emotions such as rage, anxiety, depression, and grief, our brain undergoes specific biochemical changes, which then affect organs throughout the body. It also makes sense that we can use mental-medicine techniques, such as meditation, mental imaging, positive expectations, and a strong will to live, to help us readjust our chemical balance and produce positive biochemical changes. These changes may even "turn up the juice" on our immune response and help protect us from cancer, infectious diseases, allergies, autoimmune diseases—even, perhaps, immune disorders such as AIDS.

## The Next Step: Putting Mental Medicine to Work

Now we come to what is clearly the most important, and exciting, part of this chapter. We've seen the strong evidence for the ways our mental set affects our physical health and we've learned something of *how* scientists think it does work. But the real question is, How is this knowledge being put to work *now,* to bring the "magic" of mental medicine to all of us?

Recent research suggests that day may not be so far away, because some practitioners aren't waiting until tomorrow—they are putting these techniques to work today. Certainly, the most publicized of these cases was what happened to Norman Cousins. Some years ago, Cousins fell ill with a mysterious and terrible disease. His doctors diagnosed it as ankylosing spondylitis, which is degenerative, crippling, and irreversible.

But Cousins didn't accept that dreary diagnosis. Instead, he created his own treatment plan, using positive imaging, laughter, and vitamin C to vanquish his wasting disease. Today, a decade later, he is alive and well and teaching on the UCLA medical faculty, his "irreversible" disease behind him.

Many have claimed that he was misdiagnosed, rather than face the fact that the medical orthodoxy cannot explain how Cousins healed himself. Yet his story speaks for itself: Where once he was gravely sick, immobilized by an obviously deteriorating condition, he is now back to full health. Cousins attributes his turn-around to his personal program of imaging, laughter, and positivism.

Of course, not everybody knows so well how to unlock his or her own powers and tools of mental medicine. But I believe that everybody does have the keys to do so. Today there are starting to be more and more practitioners within—and outside of—the medical community who are willing to look at how we teach people to use the tools of mental medicine to keep themselves healthy.

At the University of Massachusetts Medical Center researchers have had significant success using mental medicine to treat a wide variety of problems, including gastrointestinal disorders, high blood pressure, chronic headaches and pain, even people with coronary bypass surgery and cancer. The program, used as a complement to traditional medical care such as chemotherapy and surgery, uses several novel meditation techniques, including visualization. Dierdre was one such case. At fifty-four she was a walking textbook of medical problems. For twenty years she had had uncontrolled blood pressure at the dangerously high level of 165/105. When she enrolled in the hospital's program, she had recently undergone heart bypass surgery, suffered from arthritis so severe she couldn't raise her arms above her shoulders, and had such chronic insomnia that she averaged only two hours of sleep nightly. After only eight weeks learning to control her mental processes, her blood pressure was down to a perfect 120/70, she slept the whole night through, and she had regained virtually complete motion in her arms and shoulders. She told her doctors, "I feel really alive for the first time in my life."

Such research, though only beginning, points clearly to the possibility that this can be a powerful self-help skill many people can employ to reinforce traditional drug and medical therapy. There is starting to be a trickle of researchers who are now finding ways to put these tools to work to relieve everything from heart disease to the common cold.

For example, a Harvard professor assembled twenty-six students who reported they were on the verge of developing a cold. He took half of them to be treated by a well-known local healer, a man possessed of considerable skill and experience in assisting people to use their own internal healing abilities. The other half got a more cursory treatment from one of the healer's assistants. The results were quite dramatic: Eighty-four percent of those who got the real healer did not come down with a cold and showed a marked increase in a particular immune-system antibody in their saliva (a key part of the body's first-line defense against cold and flu germs). Of the other group, virtually the same proportion of subjects *did* come down with a cold and showed much lower levels of the immune factor in their saliva.

The same Harvard researcher also discovered what he calls the Mother Teresa Effect. He showed to a class of undergraduates a film of Mother Teresa's charity work caring for the sick and dying in Calcutta. About half were consciously inspired by her acts, the other half found the film "too religious" or "fake" and were turned off. But again, he found that samples of their saliva taken before and after the film showed a marked increase in the same immune components. Interestingly, the students' salivary immune antibodies rose regardless of how the person consciously felt about Mother Teresa. The researcher explains that the students "were still responding to the strength of her tender loving care" (Joan Z. Borysenko, "Healing

Motives: Interview with David C. McClelland," *Advances,* Institute for the Advancement of Health, Vol. 2, No. 2, Spring 1985, p. 29).

Such tender, loving care may well turn out to be a basic component of mental medicine. A British study found that heart attack patients cared for at home by the family did no worse than those cared for in a hospital cardiac intensive care unit. The researchers theorize that the "emotional strains of being moved to an intensive care unit, subjected to its atmosphere of crisis and turmoil, counterbalances the technical advantages" (Jerome Frank, *op. cit.*) But it is equally possible that the much higher level of loving, quality care provided by family members helps mobilize mental healing agents that go untapped in the hospital.

Sometimes the tools of mental medicine are so simple as to seem almost self-evident. One study gave half of the elderly residents of a nursing home the opportunity to take a more active role in their care, make decisions about their entertainment, and take care of their own room and plants. The other residents were told what to do and when and were told that the staff would "take care of everything." Researchers found that the "take-control" group became more alert and active, participated more in activities, and showed a significant improvement in well-being compared with the patients for whom the nursing home staff did everything.

A similar nursing-home study, conducted in Sweden, showed that "when elderly patients in a convalescent hospital were offered a variety of stimulating classes and social activities, their immune function improved, they had fewer infections." Even more remarkably, they *actually gained up to three-quarters of an inch in height!*

In our own country, doctors tried such an approach at a long-term veteran's hospital. When the program began, there were 289 men who had been hospitalized for between three and ten years with chronic neurologic diseases. Most had been abandoned by families, and few had any hope of ever leaving the hospital. Then the hospital brought in a rehabilitation team to get to know patients as individuals, provide group activities to reduce isolation, institute morale-boosting activities, and help social workers connect the patients to families, prospective employers, and others in the community.

The results were little short of phenomenal. Seventy percent of the patients were able to leave the hospital to rejoin their communities. Of those, 40 percent were able to become fully self-supporting, functioning members of society. Again, it seems obvious. Simply providing these people with tender, loving care allowed them to engage their own power to make themselves well. What the program really did was provide these hopeless patients with a stiff dose of positive mental medicine.

## Fighting Cancer with Pictures

When it comes to the techniques of mental medicine, we are still very much at the beginning stages. Today, although each practitioner uses slightly different means, many of these treatments are based on a process called imaging. It usually includes first relaxing, then thinking positive, concrete images, so that you can imagine, or "visualize" your goals very strongly. For some people, it is meaningful to combine their visualizations with prayer. Others use positive health-affirming statements, called affirmations. They repeat again and again: "I am feeling better," "My body is growing stronger each day," or "I feel my tumor shrinking away into nothing."

Whichever specific technique people use, all are based on the same guiding philosophy: that each of us possesses hidden innate abilities to improve our health and well-being. Unlocking these abilities helps us mobilize powerful energies for being well.

Certainly one of the most talked about, and most controversial, applications of mental medicine involves the work of the famous Simonton couple in Texas. He is a

radiation oncologist, she a psychiatric social worker. Together they have pioneered a system for encouraging patients to visualize their own immune system fighting off
cancer cells. The system, using a series of personalized
imagery conceived by the patients, is credited with several
quite dramatic remissions of late-stage cancers and is generally regarded to improve the quality of life for those who
practice it. The Simontons are the first to admit that the
treatment is not a panacea, and they recommend, as I do,
that any such program be used in addition to, not instead
of, traditional treatments. But still, their work has proved
to be a model for others interested in experimenting with
imagery and meditation to fight cancer. One such program
is in place at George Washington University. There a neu-
roimmunologist worked with ten cancer patients. They
found that by using a strict regime of imagery, patients
were actually able to increase the patients' counts of T-
lymphocytes, a crucial arm of the immune system necessary to fight cancer. An anecdotal case history, reported
by a psychiatrist at the Washington School of Psychiatry,
treated only one patient. It found that during the time he
was using imagery, bone scans revealed diminished spread
of the cancer. When he didn't, the count of his immune
cells and immune-activating hormone dropped.

Cancer is by no means the only serious disease for which
mental medicine has been tried—and has worked. The
British journal *The Lancet* reports a study in which fourteen people with high blood pressure tried relaxation and
meditation techniques to relax. Their blood pressures
dropped from an average of 145/91 to an average 135/87.
A similar study done at the same time showed similar
results with a larger group of patients. Also in *The Lancet*,
British physicians report success using meditation techniques to reduce the frequency of heart rhythm abnormal-
ities in eight out of eleven patients tested.

In our own country, the prestigious Menninger Clinic
in Topeka, Kansas, pioneered the use of biofeedback machines to teach patients to actually control their body's

internal processes. There, and in many other clinics nationwide, biofeedback has become recognized as a successful technique for lowering blood pressure and avoiding the crippling pain of migraine headaches.

A particularly interesting contemporary application of mental medicine crossed by desk today, just as I was putting the finishing touches on this chapter. For a year, a physician researcher from Vanderbilt University Medical Center has been keeping track of how long patients took to recover from minor outpatient surgery. From data derived from a preoperative questionnaire, he discovered that the best predictor of how long a patient would take to recover *was the person's own image of how long recovery would take.* That is, patients who had doubts, anxiety, fear, or misinformation before surgery generally took longer to get better afterward—independent of the operation. In effect, they had "programmed" themselves to heal slowly. Knowing this, he now recommends that doctors take more time ahead of operations to explain, reassure, and counsel preoperative patients. That way we help our patients reprogram their mental state—away from illness and *toward* a more rapid recovery.

## Try It Yourself

The fact is that, in the field of mental medicine, tomorrow is rapidly approaching. Researchers, private doctors, and patients alike are finding that mental images, programming, and expectations—what I term the tapes we play over and over again in our thoughts—can be helpful, specific means for controlling our health. For all of us, the next step is obvious: Recruit the very systems that aggravate stress and cause disease to eliminate those same diseases.

To give you an idea of the many ways you can use mental medicine in your life every day, I have included a sample meditation-imaging sequence you may want to try. You can use it to help focus your energies for better health, to reduce tension, and to help you solve problems. These basic principles were developed by a leader in the imaging field, José Silva:

1. You must *continuously desire,* believe, and expect the event or state to take place. ("My high blood pressure will become normal.")
2. You cannot create a problem.
3. *Relax* two or three times daily, sitting quietly each time for ten to fifteen minutes in a comfortable chair, your feet on the ground. With your eyes closed, put your desired mental image on an imaginary movie screen in front of you.
4. *Create* your own internal "movie" of how you want the event or situation to be—your cancer shrinking and disappearing, your blood pressure staying level in all situations, your breathing being deep and forceful.
5. *Energize* the mental image in order to trigger your body's own healing powers. To do so, repeat twenty times in succession, twice daily, an affirmation such as: "I feel myself getting better, stronger, and healthier every day. I have only positive thoughts or assumptions, and these have an effect on every aspect of my life."
6. Open your eyes, smile, and stretch.

I tell my patients to repeat this three times a day—morning, noon, and evening—for best results. I also stress that such techniques are a supplement to, not a substitute for, proven clinical treatments. They can be used hand-in-hand with traditional methods, drugs, and surgery to help us tap our own inborn healing powers, and they can help us better withstand traditional medical treatments.

If you have an illness or are under a physician's care, it is vital that you continue your prescribed therapy in concert with mental-medicine techniques. Then perhaps, as your symptoms begin to decrease, you and your doctor will be able gradually to tailor the medical and drug treatments you take and thus avoid the possibility of overtreatment. Under the supervision of your physician, you should continue to use visualizations two or three times daily.

## A Long Way to Go

We have just spent a chapter reviewing scores of studies, research findings, and experiments charting ever deeper and more profound links between mind and body than we ever thought possible. Beyond anecdotal, or even experimental, evidence, we have seen that we are gaining our first concrete, provable glimpses into the mechanics of how our brains and bodies work together to make us sick or keep us well.

I wish I could close this chapter, and this book, by saying that these findings have been wholeheartedly embraced by the medical community. They haven't. Only last year I came across the following quote in the editorial page of one of our nation's most respected medical journals, the *New England Journal of Medicine:* "It is time to acknowledge that our belief in disease as a direct reflection of mental state is largely folklore." The editorial was part of an ongoing discussion in their pages about the role that emotions and mental factors play in diseases such as heart attacks and cancer.

When I read this editorial, I have to admit, I was stunned. It's amazing, sometimes, just how much the tradition-bound medical establishment still has to learn. The kind of studies we have seen here are easily available to every member of the scientific, medical, or even interested lay public. Given the weight of all this evidence, I cannot help but feel that an editorial like the one I read is seriously behind the times. From my own vantage point, from the thousands of patients I have seen in my own medical practice, and from speaking with doctors and patients across the country, I believe that we know more than ever about many definite—and promising—avenues of how the brain can heal the body.

Nor am I alone. A fellow psychiatrist, giving a commencement address to a recent class at Johns Hopkins Medical School, put it well: "Western medicine has long recognized that emotions . . . can exacerbate such illnesses as tuberculosis, diabetes, asthma, peptic ulcer, ulcerative colitis, headache, and diseases of the cardiovascular system. But in treating these conditions we still pay inadequate attention to their psychological components."

So why, if the field of psychoneuroimmunology holds such promise, does it remain so underresearched and so controversial? In part, it is a sad fact that this field simply has not received the attention it deserves because of the high-tech, mega-bucks way we practice medicine in this country. In our system it is damnably difficult for findings to be accepted unless they derive from complicated, epidemiologically controlled protocols, statistically verified on large numbers of subjects. The advantage is that such a system helps assure top-quality medical information. The disadvantage, of course, is that it blocks new and controversial findings for years.

Another factor also conspires to keep such techniques out of the medical mainstream: It is "too simple"—any of us can do it, and we already have the tools. No large corporation or pharmaceutical manufacturer stands to make a lot of money from drug patents, fancy electronic devices, or new surgical tools. So, by the game rules of profit-motive medicine, there is scant incentive to pursue the large-scale research that would be necessary in order to prove or disprove these techniques. It is an irony that because the tools of mental medicine are so radical, so new, and yet so sensible, they have not yet received the full attention they merit. Indeed, I wish the medical community would ask, Since these are so innovative yet simple and since they pose no real medical risks whatsoever, is it not our professional duty to explore them as fully as possible without delay?

Although predictions are dangerous in medicine, I will go out on a limb: I believe that the medical profession will have to—and indeed is, slowly—broadening its outlook on the field of mental medicine. To quote a journal article from a faculty physician at Johns Hopkins Medical School, ''We are entering a period in which a holistic conception of illness and healing is gaining ever wider acceptance.''

The good news is that it does feel to me that the most enlightened and innovative medical minds are becoming increasingly open to what many of us have long believed: that it is time for our healers to add the techniques of mental medicine to our traditional stethoscopes, scalpels, and drugs. Who knows? Tomorrow's medical office may rely as much on meditation as on medication.

## Looking Back, Looking Ahead

Together, we have come to a fitting end to this book. Over the last few hundred pages we have seen that there is still a huge amount that our best medical minds don't know. This fact holds true at the frontiers of mental medicine, with the promise of progress in psychoneuroimmunology, and we have seen it is just as true for the clinically recognized, but too-often-overlooked phantom diseases.

For my part, it is my most sincere wish that you never forget how much we still have to learn—all of us. Because keeping that in mind may mean the difference between a healthy, happy, productive life and one marred and undermined by disease and ill health.

Having read this book, you have given yourself the tools to take a more active, involved role in your own well-being. You have the information to work hand-in-hand with your health care providers to make sure you get the best, most informed medical care possible.

I believe we are all on the threshold of a terrifically exciting new approach to disease treatment and prevention. I also know that it is up to all of us—me, your doctor, and *you*—to make that come true.

Good luck and good health, always.

# Index

Achromycin, 125
Acupuncture, 289
Acyclovir, 256
Adenoviruses, 254–255
Aerobic exercise program, 175, 227–228
Affirmations, 308
AIDS (autoimmune deficiency syndrome), 10, 212, 230–231, 239, 248, 254
 CMV and, 253
 medical insurance and, 53
 mental medicine and, 304
 PCC infections and, 120–121
Alcohol, 222, 228
 hypoglycemia and, 181, 184, 193–194
Alerting reaction, 172–173
Alzheimer's disease, 53
Ambulatory cardiac monitoring, 155–156
American Academy of Allergy, 113
American Academy of Sciences, 158

American Association for the Advancement of Science, 10
American Cancer Society, 296
American College of Allergy, 268
*American Family Physician*, 201–202
 on PMS incidence, 203
American Heart Association, 164, 168
 heart-healthy diet recommendations of, 158
 on regular physical checkups, 156
 scientific findings on SMI, 145–146
*American Journal of Clinical Nutrition*, 103–104
*American Journal of Epidemiology*, 22
*American Journal of Medicine*, 144–145, 152–153
*American Journal of Public Health*
 on cost of hypertension drugs, 176–177
 on PMS-caffeine link, 219